Practical Aspects of Cognitive Impairment and the Dementias

Editors

PHILIP B. GORELICK
FARZANEH A. SOROND

CLINICS IN GERIATRIC MEDICINE

www.geriatric.theclinics.com

February 2023 • Volume 39 • Number 1

ELSEVIER

1600 John F. Kennedy Boulevard • Suite 1800 • Philadelphia, Pennsylvania, 19103-2899

http://www.theclinics.com

CLINICS IN GERIATRIC MEDICINE Volume 39, Number 1
February 2023 ISSN 0749–0690, ISBN-13: 978-0-323-96069-4

Editor: Taylor Hayes
Developmental Editor: Hannah Almira Lopez

Clinics in Geriatric Medicine (ISSN 0749-0690) is published quarterly by Elsevier Inc., 360 Park Avenue South, New York, NY 10010-1710. Months of issue are February, May, August, and November. Business and Editorial Offices: 1600 John F. Kennedy Blvd., Suite 1800, Philadelphia, PA 191023-2899. Periodicals postage paid at New York, NY, and additional mailing offices. Subscription prices are $312.00 per year (US individuals), $748.00 per year (US institutions), $100.00 per year (US & Canadian student/resident), $340.00 per year (Canadian individuals), $946.00 per year (Canadian institutions), $444.00 per year (international individuals), $946.00 per year (international institutions), and $195.00 per year (international student/resident). Foreign air speed delivery is included in all *Clinics* subscription prices. All prices are subject to change without notice. POSTMASTER: Send address changes to *Clinics in Geriatric Medicine,* Elsevier Health Sciences Division, Subscription Customer Service, 3251 Riverport Lane, Maryland Heights, MO 63043. **Telephone: 1-800-654-2452 (U.S. and Canada); 314-447-8871 (outside U.S. and Canada). Fax: 314-447-8029. E-mail:** journalscustomerservice-usa@elsevier.com **(for print support) or** journalsonlinesupport-usa@elsevier.com **(for online support).**

Reprints. For copies of 100 or more, of articles in this publication, please contact the Commercial Reprints Department, Elsevier Inc., 360 Park Avenue South, New York, New York 10010-1710. Tel.: 212-633-3874; Fax: 212-633-3820, E-mail: reprints@elsevier.com.

Clinics in Geriatric Medicine is covered in *MEDLINE/PubMed (Index Medicus), EMBASE/Excerpta Medica, Current Contents/Clinical Medicine (CC/CM),* and the *Cumulative Index to Nursing & Allied Health Literature.*

Contributors

EDITORS

PHILIP B. GORELICK, MD, MPH
Professor, The Ken and Ruth Davee Department of Neurology, Northwestern University Feinberg School of Medicine, Adjunct Professor of Neurology, Department of Neurology, Division of Stroke, Northwestern University, Chicago, Illinois, USA

FARZANEH A. SOROND, MD, PhD
Associate Dean for Faculty Development, Vice Chair for Faculty Development and Education, Department of Neurology, Chief of Stroke and Neurocritical Care in the Department of Neurology, Dean Richard H. Young and Ellen Stearns Young Professor, Professor of Neurology (Stroke) and Neurology (Neurocritical Care), Northwestern University Feinberg School of Medicine, Chicago, Illinois, USA

AUTHORS

SHEENA BARATONO, MD, PhD
Cognitive Neurology Unit, Beth Israel Deaconess Medical Center, Brookline, Massachusetts, USA

ALESSANDRO BIFFI, MD
Department of Neurology, Massachusetts General Hospital, Harvard Medical School, Henry and Allison McCance Center for Brain Health, Boston, Massachusetts, USA

BORNA BONAKDARPOUR, MD, FAAN
Mesulam Center for Cognitive Neurology and Alzheimer's Disease, The Ken and Ruth Davee Department of Neurology, Northwestern University Feinberg School of Medicine Chicago, Illinois, USA

SCOTT E. COUNTS, PhD
Departments of Translational Neuroscience and Family Medicine, Michigan State University, Hauenstein Neuroscience Center, Mercy Health Saint Mary's Medical Center, Grand Rapids, Michigan, USA

JOHN D. CRAWFORD, PhD
Centre for Healthy Brain Ageing, University of New South Wales, Sydney, New South Wales, Australia

VICTOR A. DEL BENE, PhD
Department of Neurology, Division of Neuropsychology, The Evelyn F. McKnight Brain Institute, University of Alabama at Birmingham Heersink School of Medicine, Birmingham, Alabama, USA

ANNE M. DORRANCE, PhD
Department of Pharmacology and Toxicology, Michigan State University, East Lansing, Michigan, USA

ADAM GERSTENECKER, PhD
Department of Neurology, Division of Neuropsychology, The Evelyn F. McKnight Brain Institute, University of Alabama at Birmingham Heersink School of Medicine, Birmingham, Alabama, USA

MAHSA GIFANI, MD
Department of Translational Neuroscience, Michigan State University, Grand Rapids, Michigan, USA

MARCIA N. GORDON, PhD
Department of Translational Neuroscience, Michigan State University, Grand Rapids, Michigan, USA

PHILIP B. GORELICK, MD, MPH
Professor, The Ken and Ruth Davee Department of Neurology, Northwestern University Feinberg School of Medicine, Adjunct Professor of Neurology, Department of Neurology, Division of Stroke, Northwestern University, Chicago, Illinois, USA

BETUL KARA, MS
Department of Translational Neuroscience, Michigan State University, Grand Rapids, Michigan, USA

BEN C.P. LAM, PhD
Centre for Healthy Brain Ageing, University of New South Wales, Sydney, New South Wales, Australia

RONALD M. LAZAR, PhD
Department of Neurology, Division of Neuropsychology, The Evelyn F. McKnight Brain Institute, Department of Neurobiology, University of Alabama at Birmingham Heersink School of Medicine, Birmingham, Alabama, USA

DARREN M. LIPNICKI, PhD
Centre for Healthy Brain Ageing, University of New South Wales, Sydney, New South Wales, Australia

SIMIN MAHINRAD, MD, PhD
Research Assistant Professor, Department of Neurology, Northwestern University Feinberg School of Medicine, Chicago, Illinois, USA

AKASHLEENA MALLICK, MD
Department of Neurology, Massachusetts General Hospital, Harvard Medical School, Henry and Allison McCance Center for Brain Health, Boston, Massachusetts, USA

RUPAL I. MEHTA, MD
Rush Alzheimer's Disease Center, Department of Pathology, Rush University Medical Center, Chicago, Illinois, USA

LOUISE MEWTON, PhD
Centre for Healthy Brain Ageing, University of New South Wales, Sydney, New South Wales, Australia

DAVID L. NYENHUIS, PhD
Associate Professor, Neuropsychology Section, Hauenstein Neuroscience Center, Mercy Health of West Michigan, Grand Rapids, Michigan, USA; Department of Psychology, LCC International University, Klaipeda, Lithuania

LANDON PERLETT, MD
Department of Clinical Neurosciences, University of Calgary, Calgary, Alberta, Canada

DANIEL PRESS, MD
Cognitive Neurology Unit, Beth Israel Deaconess Medical Center, Brookline, Massachusetts, USA

JACLYN RECKOW, PhD
Neuropsychology Section, Hauenstein Neuroscience Center, Mercy Health of West Michigan, Grand Rapids, Michigan, USA

BEHNAM SABAYAN, MD, PhD
Department of Neurology, HealthPartners Neuroscience Center, St Paul, Minnesota, USA; Division of Epidemiology and Community Health, School of Public Health, University of Minnesota, Minneapolis, Minnesota, USA

PERMINDER S. SACHDEV, MD, PhD
Centre for Healthy Brain Ageing, University of New South Wales, Neuropsychiatric Institute, The Prince of Wales Hospital, Sydney, New South Wales, Australia

JULIE A. SCHNEIDER, MD, MS
Rush Alzheimer's Disease Center, Department of Pathology, Department of Neurological Sciences, Rush University Medical Center, Chicago, Illinois, USA

SANAZ SEDAGHAT, PhD
Division of Epidemiology and Community Health, School of Public Health, University of Minnesota, Minneapolis, Minnesota, USA

ERIC E. SMITH, MD, MPH
Department of Clinical Neurosciences, University of Calgary, Calgary, Alberta, Canada

FARZANEH A. SOROND, MD, PhD
Associate Dean for Faculty Development, Vice Chair for Faculty Development and Education, Department of Neurology, Chief of Stroke and Neurocritical Care in the Department of Neurology, Dean Richard H. Young and Ellen Stearns Young Professor, Professor of Neurology (Stroke) and Neurology (Neurocritical Care), Northwestern University Feinberg School of Medicine, Chicago, Illinois, USA

CLARA TAKARABE, CMP
Mesulam Center for Cognitive Neurology and Alzheimer's Disease, The Ken and Ruth Davee Department of Neurology, Northwestern University Feinberg School of Medicine, Chicago, Illinois, USA

KATHRYN A. WYMAN-CHICK, PsyD
Department of Neurology, HealthPartners Neuroscience Center, St Paul, Minnesota, USA

Contents

Epidemiology of Cognitive Impairment and the Dementias

> Dementia spectrum disorders (DSDs) are a major cause of mortality and disability worldwide. DSDs encompass a large group of medical conditions that all ultimately lead to major functional and cognitive decline and disability. Demographic and comorbid conditions that are associated with DSDs have significant prognostic and preventive implications. In this article, we will discuss the global and regional burden of DSDs and cover key demographic and clinical conditions linked with DSDs. In the absence of disease-modifying treatments, the role of primary prevention has become more prominent. Implementation of preventive measures requires an understanding of predisposing and exacerbating factors.

Establishing a Diagnosis of Cognitive Impairment and Dementia

> Elderly patients and their families are concerned about the patients' cognitive abilities, and cognitive screening is an efficient diagnostic tool, as long as clinicians administer the screens in a standardized manner and interpret the screen results accurately. The following brief summary reviews commonly used screening instruments and provides information about how to interpret screening test results. It concludes by showing how cognitive screening fits into a four-step process (Education, Screening, Follow-up, and Referral) of how to respond to patients with cognitive concerns.

> Neuropsychologists evaluate patients for cognitive decline and dementia, using validated psychometric tests, along with behavioral observation, record review, clinical interview, and information about psychological functioning, to evaluate brain–behavior relationships and aid in differential diagnosis and treatment planning. Also considered are premorbid functioning, education, sex, socioeconomic status, primary language, culture, and race-related health disparities when selecting tests, interpreting performance, and providing a diagnostic impression. Neuropsychologists

Underlying Neuropathology and Basic Mechanisms

inclusions (ie, proteinopathies) but other brain abnormalities are also related to dementia. Beta-amyloid and tau aggregates are hallmarks of AD. Other tissue substrates include Lewy bodies, TDP-43 inclusions, vascular brain lesions, and mixed pathologies. This review highlights the complexity of neurodegenerative and other disease substrates and summarizes topography of these lesions and concepts of mixed brain pathologies, resistance, and resilience.

Aging, familial gene mutations, and genetic, environmental, and modifiable lifestyle risk factors predispose individuals to cognitive impairment or dementia by influencing the efficacy of multiple, often interdependent cellular and molecular homeostatic pathways mediating neuronal, glial, and vascular integrity and, ultimately, cognitive status. This review summarizes data from foundational and recent breakthrough studies to highlight common and differential vascular and nonvascular pathogenic mechanisms underlying the progression of Alzheimer disease, vascular dementia, frontotemporal dementia, and dementia with Lewy bodies.

Prevention and Treatment of Common Forms of Cognitive Impairment and Dementia

One of the most challenging clinical expressions of population aging is cognitive impairment and dementia. Among risk factors for the development of dementia, modifiable vascular risk factors have emerged as contributors to both vascular and nonvascular types of dementia. Epidemiologic studies have been particularly informative in understanding the link between vascular risks and dementia across the life course. We discuss vascular risks for dementia and cognitive impairment and practical management recommendations.

Ideally, dementia care should be provided by a collaborative team. Eligible patients should be treated with the cognitive-enhancing medications, the cholinesterase inhibitors and memantine. For most of the common causes of dementia, there are no disease-modifying medications, with the exception that vascular dementia can be prevented by treating vascular risk factors to prevent stroke. There is hope that Alzheimer disease can be treated by using monoclonal antibodies that target amyloid beta, although more trials are needed. Holistic, patient-centered care can enhance quality and extend the time that the patient can live safely in the community.

> In the absence of effective treatments for dementia, maintaining cognitive health in old age is one of the major challenges facing aging societies. Interventions for cognitive health that are tailored to the person are more likely to bring the best benefits with a minimum burden. We review the existing literature on this topic and discuss the role of the primary care physician.

Beyond Memory and Other Cognitive Dysfunction: Neurobehavioral and Psychiatric Disorders

> Neurobehavioral and neuropsychiatric symptoms are highly prevalent among individuals diagnosed with cognitive impairment or dementia and impact the quality of life for patients and caregivers alike. Diagnosis and management of these conditions (including primarily depression, anxiety, apathy, psychosis, agitation, and aggression) is crucial to optimal patient care outcomes in clinical practice. The present article provides a practical review of diagnostic approaches and management strategies for behavioral and neuropsychiatric disorders arising in patients with cognitive impairment, up to and including dementia.

Working Together Globally

> Understanding dementia and cognitive impairment is a global effort needing data from multiple sources across diverse ethno-regional groups. Methodological heterogeneity means that these data often require harmonization to make them comparable before analysis. We discuss the benefits and challenges of harmonization, both retrospective and prospective, broadly and with a focus on data types that require particular sorts of approaches, including neuropsychological test scores and neuroimaging data. Throughout our discussion, we illustrate general principles and give examples of specific approaches in the context of contemporary research in dementia and cognitive impairment from around the world.

CLINICS IN GERIATRIC MEDICINE

FORTHCOMING ISSUES

May 2023
Geriatric Dental Medicine
Joseph M. Calabrese and
Michelle M. Henshaw, *Editors*

August 2023
Updates in Palliative Care
Kimberly Curseen, *Editor*

RECENT ISSUES

November 2022
Polypharmacy
Edward L. Schneider and
Brandon K. Koretz, *Editors*

August 2022
COVID-19 in the Geriatric Patient
Francesco Landi, *Editor*

ISSUES OF RELATED INTEREST

Primary Care: Clinics in Office Practice
https://www.primarycare.theclinics.com/
Psychiatric Clinics
http://www.psych.theclinics.com/
Neurologic Clinics
http://www.neurologic.theclinics.com/

THE CLINICS ARE AVAILABLE ONLINE!
Access your subscription at:
www.theclinics.com

Preface

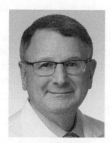 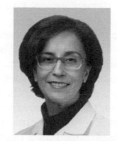

Philip B. Gorelick, MD, MPH   Farzaneh A. Sorond, MD, PhD
Editors

During the past 40 years, we have witnessed a substantial transformation of the dementia landscape. Once thought to be largely a consequence of "cerebrovascular insufficiency," the dementias later became recognized as a group of disorders predominantly characterized as neurodegenerative in nature, with Alzheimer disease (AD) being the leading cause. In the 1990s, fueled by Decade of the Brain legislation in the United States, there was a concerted effort to better understand AD and its key underlying neuropathologic manifestations: neuronal death, neurofibrillary tangles, and amyloid plaques. The domination of the research field by AD studies during this time period led some pundits to claim the field had been "Alzheimerized." However, by the late 1990s and early 2000s, it was becoming apparent based on epidemiologic studies that vascular risks (e.g. hypertension, diabetes mellitus, and other factors) were possible risks not only for cognitive impairment associated with stroke but also for AD. A renewed emphasis on vascular risks as precursors of cognitive impairment and dementia led to an evolution and refinement of diagnostic terminology used to categorize vascular forms of cognitive impairment. The term multi-infarct dementia, coined in the 1970s, was replaced by vascular dementia, which was later superseded by vascular cognitive impairment or vascular cognitive disorders. The latter two terms are now commonly used by clinical experts to refer to dementia or cognitive impairment associated with stroke. Parenthetically, and more recently, there has been a movement to replace the time-honored term "dementia." In fact, the *Diagnostic and Statistical Manual of Mental Disorders* (Fifth Edition) now refers to "major or mild neurocognitive disorder" rather than using the term "dementia."

Initially, there was hesitancy by the AD research community to embrace the possible role of vascular risks as precursor factors for the dementias. Over time, however, the concept of prevention of the dementias through modification of vascular risks gained traction in clinical practice. Whereas AD has played a dominant role in the clinical landscape of the dementias, research breakthroughs in regards to the potential importance of vascular risks as precursors to age-related cognitively impairing disorders, and community necropsy studies showing the importance of "mixed" neuropathologic

Clin Geriatr Med 39 (2023) xiii–xv
https://doi.org/10.1016/j.cger.2022.08.005
0749-0690/23/© 2022 Published by Elsevier Inc.

geriatric.theclinics.com

changes (e.g. cooccurrence of stroke and AD brain changes) in more than 50% of the patients, provide support for the importance of vascular risk factors and cerebrovascular disease in the genesis of the dementias. Vascular risks provide an important opportunity for prevention of the dementias, as traditional vascular risk factors are preventable and modifiable.

Our understanding of neurocognitive disorders has substantially advanced largely in part due to an evolution in neuroimaging. Springboarded by the *Human Connectome Project*, our knowledge of brain structure and function has been greatly enhanced by the following neuroimaging techniques: diffusion tensor imaging, functional MRI, cerebral blood flow, and neuroreceptor density elucidation. Such techniques have been complemented by advanced genetic and blood and cerebrospinal fluid biomarker discovery. Furthermore, the estimated 100 billion neurons of the brain are now conceptualized as a network of key neuronal hubs with local and more far-reaching connections. The strength of connectivity within and between the brain networks helps to determine brain function and potential for resilience and resistance to cerebral injury. In addition, the white matter of the brain, an important highway connecting various regions of the brain, now serves as a target for prevention and treatment efforts to preserve cerebral structure and function, and thus, cognition.

In this issue of *Clinics in Geriatric Medicine*, we provide six sections geared to the primary care geriatrician, other primary care clinicians, allied health care workers in the field, and researchers on practical aspects of cognitive impairment and the dementias. Section 1 is devoted to the epidemiology of neurocognitive disorders and the dementias, and how common these disorders are worldwide. Section 2 discusses how to establish a diagnosis and includes information on selection and interpretation of cognitive screening tests and formal neuropsychologic tests, neuroimaging aspects from a clinician's perspective, the role of blood and cerebrospinal fluid biomarkers, and a case-based approach to establishing a diagnosis of cognitive impairment and dementia by underlying subtype. Section 3 emphasizes neuropathologic findings and underlying mechanisms of cognitively impairing disorders. Section 4 reviews the role of vascular risk factors and treatment and introduces the concepts of brain resistance and resilience and how cognitive reserve may determine risk and outcome. Section 5 discusses the diagnosis of neuropsychiatric and behavioral aspects of the dementias, and Section 6 provides a research perspective on data harmonization as we work globally to end the scourge of neurocognitive disorders and the dementias.

Geriatricians and other primary health care providers frequently encounter patients in practice in need of cognitive assessment and comprehensive management. The articles compiled in this issue of *Clinics in Geriatric Medicine* provide guidance in these areas. In addition, with the recognition of vascular risks as targets for prevention of cognitive impairment and dementia, geriatricians and other primary health care providers are now in a lead position to manage such factors. The *American Heart Association* (AHA) previously identified three vascular health behaviors (diet, physical activity, nicotine exposure/smoking) and four vascular health factors (body weight, blood lipids, blood glucose, and blood pressure), referred to as *Life's Simple 7* (LS7), as targets for preservation of brain health. Recently, AHA added an eighth factor, sleep health (7 to <9 hours per day of sleep), to the list of target factors, and renamed LS7, *Life's Essential 8*. By prevention and treatment of vascular risks, we hope to prevent or delay neurocognitive disorders that affect millions of persons worldwide. As scientific discovery advances, it is hoped we will soon be able to utilize biomarkers to provide individualized and targeted preventatives and treatments for those at risk of or who have neurocognitive disorders.

Philip B. Gorelick, MD, MPH
Davee Department of Neurology
Northwestern University Feinberg School of Medicine
635 N. Michigan Avenue
Chicago, IL 60611, USA

Farzaneh A. Sorond, MD, PhD
Department of Neurology
Northwestern University
Feinberg School of Medicine
420 East Superior Street
Chicago, IL 60611, USA

E-mail addresses:
philip.gorelick@gmail.com (P.B. Gorelick)
Farzaneh.Sorond@nm.org (F.A. Sorond)

Epidemiology of Cognitive Impairment and the Dementias

The Burden of Dementia Spectrum Disorders and Associated Comorbid and Demographic Features

Behnam Sabayan, MD, PhD[a,b],*, Kathryn A. Wyman-Chick, PsyD[a],
Sanaz Sedaghat, PhD[b]

KEYWORDS

• Dementia • Comorbidity • Biological sex • Race • Ethnicity

KEY POINTS

• The dementia spectrum disorders represent a wide range of pathophysiological processes that all ultimately lead to major functional and cognitive decline and disability.
• With the population aging, and in the absence of disease-modifying treatment, preventive strategies are key to decrease the burden of dementia spectrum disorders.
• Biological sex, race, and ethnicity in combination with various demographic and clinical factors act in concert to change the probability of developing dementia spectrum disorders and influence the prognosis.

BACKGROUND

Dementia spectrum disorders (DSDs) are a large group of medical conditions with a wide range of pathophysiological processes which all ultimately lead to major functional and cognitive decline and disability.[1] Currently, more than 55 million people live with DSDs worldwide, and there are nearly 10 million new cases every year.[2] Alzheimer's disease (AD) is the most common form of DSDs accounting for 60% to 70% of cases.[3] Although previously it was thought that AD is a pure neurodegenerative entity due to the accumulation of amyloid plaques and neurofibrillary tangles, there is increasing evidence showing that most of AD cases have mixed pathologies and multiple pathophysiological processes interact with each other.[4] AD neuropathology is not only a mixed proteinopathy (amyloid and tau) but also, in more than half of

[a] Department of Neurology, HealthPartners Neuroscience Center, 295 Phalen Boulevard, St Paul, MN 55130, USA; [b] Division of Epidemiology and Community Health, School of Public Health, University of Minnesota, 1300 S Second Street, Suite 300, Minneapolis, MN 55454, USA
* Corresponding author.
E-mail address: bsabayan@umn.edu

Clin Geriatr Med 39 (2023) 1–14
https://doi.org/10.1016/j.cger.2022.07.001
0749-0690/23/© 2022 Elsevier Inc. All rights reserved.

geriatric.theclinics.com

cases, has overlap with cerebrovascular pathologies and Lewy body disease.[5] In terms of frequency, AD is followed by vascular dementia (VaD), Lewy body dementia (LBD), and frontotemporal dementia (FTD). Approximately 5% of DSD cases remain undifferentiated, frequently because of mixed features.[6] Given the accumulating data showing a large overlap of neuropathologies across different dementia subtypes and the spectrum of clinical presentations, even within a specific subtype, the utility of clinical subtype designations needs to be further investigated.[7]

Aging is the main driver and common determinant for the incidence of DSDs. In the vast majority of cases, the prevalence of individual dementia conditions is age-dependent. With the current worldwide trends in population aging and the increase of life expectancy, the number of patients with DSDs has significantly increased.[8] It is expected that the number of patients with DSDs will nearly triple worldwide by 2050 imposing a major financial toll on health care systems and primary caregivers.[9] Despite this alarming increase in the burden of DSDs, currently there are no therapeutics or disease-modifying treatments available. This mismatch calls for better recognition of DSD risk factors and the developing of effective preventive measures that delay disease onset and slow down the progress of the disease when DSDs are in their prodromal phase. In this review, we will provide an overview of global and regional burden of DSDs and will discuss the roles of primary and secondary prevention strategies. In addition, we will focus on sex, ethnicity, and race in relation to the individual occurrence of DSDs and outcomes.

BURDEN OF DEMENTIA SPECTRUM DISORDERS

Despite increased awareness and several international efforts to decrease the burden of dementia, DSDs have remained a major cause of mortality and disability worldwide. The number of patients with DSDs is estimated to have increased by more than 100% between 1990 and 2016, largely due to population aging and improvement in diagnosis and early recognition of DSD cases.[10] Several reports from European countries and North America have shown that the incidence of DSDs is decreasing in those regions. Nonetheless, a major disparity exists in this pattern.[11] Even within large countries, such as the United States, various trends are observed. In 2019, there were 57.4 million individuals living with DSDs globally. The Global Burden of Diseases (GBD) study showed that about 26 million people will be added to this patient group by 2030 and it is forecasted that the number will consistently rise to more than 150 million individuals in 2050.[9]

The societal cost of DSDs is substantial. In 2019, the estimated total global societal cost of dementia was US$ 1.3 trillion, and these costs are expected to surpass US$ 2.8 trillion by 2030 as both the number of people living with dementia and care costs increase.[12] In addition to the direct costs, burden on family members and caregivers is significant and it is estimated that about 50% of the global cost of dementia is attributed to informal care.[13]

There will be a rapid surge in the number of patients with DSDs in developing countries. Current estimates indicate that more than two-thirds of patients with DSDs live in low- and middle-income countries.[14] There are multiple reasons behind a surge in the number of DSD patients in low- and middle-income countries. First, populations are rapidly aging in those countries. By 2050%, 80% of all older people will live in low- and middle-income countries.[15] Second, although the burden of communicable diseases has significantly decreased globally, the incidence and prevalence of non-communicable conditions (in particular cerebrovascular risk factors such as hypertension [HTN] and diabetes) are rapidly increasing in low- and middle-income countries.[16]

It has been consistently shown that exposure to vascular risk factors and covert cerebrovascular injuries in middle age are strongly associated with DSDs in older age.[17] Third, apart from risk factors, comorbidities associated with DSDs are on the rise in those regions as well. As we and others have shown in the past, impaired kidney function, coronary artery disease, and heart failure are all independently linked with future risk of cognitive impairment and development of DSDs.[18] Limited resources and infrastructure for dementia care in low- and middle-income countries is another major challenge and can lead to political and societal instability in those regions.[19]

THE ROLE OF PRIMARY PREVENTION

DSDs for a long time have been considered as progressive and neurodegenerative processes without available opportunities to prevent them or change the course of the disease.[20] Over the last decades, our understanding of DSDs has significantly changed. It is now well-established that the in most cases of DSDs, we are encountering multiple pathologies that can provide the chance to modify disease course from various angles.[21] An increasing number of observational evidence has shown that a midlife positive lifestyle profile is closely related to a delayed onset of DSDs.[22] Such studies have consistently shown that cardiovascular risk factors, inactivity and poor sleep quantity and quality predict an accelerated cognitive decline and higher future risk of DSDs. Such observational data provide a basis for implementing public health and individual level measures that change the risk exposure from a younger age and delay the onset and progression of cognitive impairment. Multiple prediction models have shown that even 1 year delay in the onset of DSDs, an, in particular, its common form AD, significantly reduces the heavy societal burden of these conditions. For instance, it is estimated that preventive strategies that delay onset of AD for 5 years will result in 41% lower prevalence and 40% lower cost of AD in 2050. A delay of AD onset by 1 year reduces the prevalence of AD (in those 70 years and older) in 2030 from 5.8 (status quo) to 4.7 million, and in 2050 from 9.1 to 7.8 million.[23]

MODIFIABLE RISK FACTORS

Available evidence indicates that about 40% of DSD cases are attributed to modifiable risk factors.[24] The magnitude of the contribution of modifiable risk factors provides a significant opportunity to decrease the risk of developing DSDs and delay the clinical onset.

Demographic and Clinical Factors

Among various modifiable risk factors, years of formal education have one of the strongest associations with future risk of DSDs.[25] Years of education represent literacy and training backgrounds and it can be a proxy for socio-demographic status and favorable early childhood and life course experiences. Education also can reflect cognitive reserve and inherent brain resilience.[26] One confounding factor in relation to the inverse association of years of education and risk of dementia is that individuals of high intellect tend to compensate for cognitive impairment symptoms which can lead to a delayed formal diagnosis of DSDs.[27]

Midlife diabetes mellitus (DM) and HTN are two other major risk factors that are strongly associated with DSD incidence. Several studies and meta-analyses have shown that DM is associated with more than 50% higher risk of DSDs.[28] It is estimated that more than 30% of older patients with DM suffer from cognitive impairment to the degrees that affect the quality of life and independence in daily activities.[29] Impaired glycemic control is detrimental to brain health and risk of cognitive impairment regardless of age.[30]

On the contrary, the relationship between HTN and DSDs is mainly age-dependent.[31] Midlife HTN is a strong and consistent risk factor for older age DSDs and cognitive impairment but low blood pressure and increased blood pressure variability can be also harmful to cognitive function in old age.[32,33] Life course data show that subjects who develop DSDs later in life have a tendency for an increased blood pressure in midlife but years to decades before full-blown dementia their blood pressure starts to decline.[34] Cardiovascular risks are further discussed in Chapter 9.

Lifestyle Factors

Lifestyle factors play key roles in the preservation of brain health and brain structural and functional integrity.[35] Physical inactivity is one of the better-established factors for cognitive impairment and incident DSDs.[36] The exact mechanism underlying the link between physical activity and cognitive function is unclear; however, several experimental, radiological, and epidemiologic studies have shown positive effects of physical activity on reducing systemic inflammation, cardiorespiratory fitness, improved cerebral blood flow, and cerebrovascular vasoreactivity.[37] Adequate and high-quality sleep is another factor that may contribute to the prevention of DSDs.[38] Basic science studies have consistently reported that high-quality sleep is needed for the clearance of brain metabolic waste products and proteins implicated in the pathogenesis of DSDs including amyloid beta.[39]

Based on several systematic reviews and meta-analyses form prospective longitudinal studies, current smoking increases the risk of cognitive decline and DSDs.[40] Smoking cessation may reduce the risk of DSDs to levels comparable to those who have not smoked but the detrimental effects of smoking might remain even after years of not smoking. A study of a large multi-ethnic cohort found that heavy smoking in middle age can double the risk of DSDs later in life.[41] Similarly, heavy alcohol use is strongly linked with future risk of DSDs.[42] There are inconsistent data on a possible positive effect of moderate drinking but this finding has not been replicated in relation to favorable brain outcomes. Current data indicate that any amount of alcohol may be harmful to the brain.[42]

Information on the effects of specific dietary elements and nutrients on reducing the risk of DSDs is limited and conflicting. Given that many elements of diet are interrelated and interactive, the idea of a whole dietary pattern approach has gained interest.[43] Various cohort studies reported that dietary patterns such as the Mediterranean diet (with limited red meat and abundance of whole grains, fruits and vegetables, fish, nuts, and olive oil) and DASH (Dietary Approaches to Stop Hypertension) or the combination (Mediterranean-DASH Intervention for Neurodegenerative Delay (MIND)) diets are strongly associated with better cerebrovascular and cognitive outcomes.[44]

Social engagement is another factor that has received a great deal of attention over the last few years.[45] There are observational studies that investigated the relationship between the degree of social engagement (through activities such as volunteer work, joining a club, and religious gathering) and risk of cognitive decline and DSDs. Overall, the evidence is consistent that engagement in those activities is associated with a lower risk of cognitive impairment. Whether social engagement itself is protective or it is an indicator of baseline physical and cognitive health is yet to be determined.[46] Regardless of the mechanism it is recommended that older adults avoid social isolation and participate in group activities that increase the sense of belonging to a community.

Medical conditions and medications. Consistent evidence from epidemiologic, experimental, and neuropathological studies indicates that traumatic brain injury (TBI) (in a dose–response fashion) in particular in older age elevates the risk of developing DSDs.[47] History of a significant TBI is associated with two to four times higher risk of DSDs and is a major factor contributing in early onset dementia in individuals without a genetic predisposition.[48] There is an increasing recognition of chronic traumatic encephalopathy (CTE), a type of dementia with distinctive clinical and pathologic features, among professional football, soccer, and hockey players.[49] However, the current data suggest that TBI-related cognitive impairment is not limited to professional sports players and it can be seen in the general population as well.[50]

Depression is another medical condition associated with future risk of cognitive decline and DSDs. The relationship between mood disorders and DSDs is complex. Mood and behavioral changes are common among a wide range of DSDs and it is likely that depression can precede cognitive symptoms as an early manifestation of brain structural and functional changes underlying DSDs.[51]

Previously, in a meta-analysis, we have shown that a history of coronary heart disease is associated with a 27% increased risk of DSDs and a history of heart failure is associated with a 60% of increased DSDs risk. It has been shown that up to 70% of older patients with end-stage renal disease have moderate to severe degrees of cognitive impairment.[52] The mechanism underlying such elevated risk is thought to be endothelial dysfunction, impaired cerebrovascular hemodynamics, and micro- and macrovascular injuries to the cerebrovascular system.[53]

Apart from medical conditions, polypharmacy and in particular use of anticholinergic medications can increase the risk of DSDs.[54,55] Medications with anticholinergic properties are frequently used in several conditions associated with aging. Examples include anticholinergic antidepressants, anti-Parkinson drugs, antipsychotics, bladder antimuscarinic medications, and antiepileptic drugs. It is highly recommended to monitor for and limit the use of such medications in geriatric populations, when feasible, to lower the risk of cognitive impairment and DSDs.

HIGH RISK AND POPULATION-BASED APPROACH IN DEMENTIA SPECTRUM DISORDER PREVENTION

Two main strategies for primary prevention of DSDs include; high-risk versus population-based approaches. The high-risk approach puts emphasis on the recognition of high-risk individuals who carry risk factors or medical conditions associated with DSDs. Case detection usually starts with an assessment by health care professionals. Treatment of HTN, diabetes, and avoiding anticholinergic medications are clear examples of this type of approach. On the contrary, a population-based approach aims to lower the average levels of exposure to risk factors, and thereby lower the incidence of DSDs at the population level.[56] Advancement of formal education, increasing awareness about HTN, and promotion of social engagement for older subjects are among the examples. Although high-risk group interventions are effective and can reduce the risk of DSDs in certain individuals, the available evidence suggests that population-based strategies can have a larger magnitude of influence. **Fig. 1** presents the concepts of high-risk versus population-based preventive strategies.

SEX DIFFERENCES IN DEMENTIA OCCURRENCE AND OUTCOMES

Table 1 summarizes sex differences in DSDs. Current data indicate that women are more than 50% at higher risk for developing DSDs.[57] There is increasing evidence to suggest that biological sex (sex chromosomes and gonadal hormones) affects

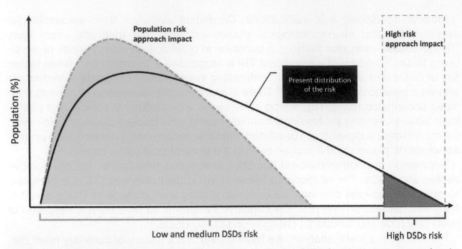

Fig. 1. The difference between high risk versus population-based preventive approaches in changing the risk distribution curve. Although the high-risk approach impacts a small number of patients in the society, the population-based approach shifts the risk distribution curve to a larger extend.

the prevalence and clinical presentation of neurodegenerative diseases.[58,59] However, gender (social, cultural, and environmental factors) may also influence the presentation of DSDs.[59]

AD is more common among women than men, particularly after age 85.[58,60,61] Women tend to have more severe cognitive deficits than men at the time of AD diagnosis and women also show faster rates of cognitive decline following an AD diagnosis. It is not clear if there are sex-specific protective factors that can delay the onset of AD. However, women perform better on tests of verbal memory throughout the lifespan, which may cause delays in AD symptom recognition and diagnosis.[62] There are also sex differences in neuropsychiatric symptoms in AD as well. Among patients diagnosed with AD, women are more likely to experience depression and delusions, although apathy is more prevalent in men.[63] Women over the age of 75 are more likely to have risk factors for VaD including diabetes, HTN, and hyperlipidemia as compared with men with similar age. Throughout their lifespan, women have specific hormonal influences that may place them at a higher risk of developing the cerebrovascular disease.[57] For example, early menopause, preeclampsia, and gestational diabetes are associated with an increased risk of future cardiovascular and cerebrovascular events.[64]

A recent large multicenter study among patients with FTD showed that there are differences in clinical phenotypes between men and women, including a higher prevalence of behavioral variant FTD in men and a higher prevalence of primary progressive aphasia (PPA) in women.[65] Women with PPA aphasia show more severe language deficits and faster rates of decline relative to men with PPA.[66] Among individuals with behavioral variant FTD, women were found to have a greater degree of frontotemporal atrophy compared with men with similar clinical presentations, suggesting a higher degree of cognitive reserve or resiliency in women.[67] Women showed fewer changes in apathy, sleep, or appetite than men with similar clinical disease stages. There does not seem to be sex differences in the rates of genetic FTD, but pooled data indicate sporadic FTD may be more prevalent among men. Researchers hypothesized this may be related to underdiagnosis among women who present with

Table 1
Brief summary of sex and race/ethnicity differences in dementia spectrum disorders

	Sex	Race/Ethnicity
Alzheimer's disease	• Greater prevalence in women after age 85 • Female APOE e4 carriers are at a higher risk of hippocampal atrophy compared with male APOE e4 carriers • Depression and delusions are more common in women, whereas apathy is more common in men	• Black and Hispanic adults in the US have higher rates of AD relative to Non-Hispanic White adults • Hispanic populations are more likely to have concomitant vascular pathology
Vascular dementia	• Early menopause, preeclampsia, and gestational diabetes are associated with increased risk of cerebrovascular disease • Women are more likely to have diabetes, hypertension, and hyperlipidemia after age 75	• The burden of cerebrovascular disease is high among Black, Hispanic, and Asian populations.
Frontotemporal dementia	• Primary Progressive Aphasia is more common in women, whereas behavioral variant is more common among men • Men are more likely to show changes in motivation, sleep, and appetite • No differences in rates of genetic FTD, but sporadic FTD may be more common in men	• The limited amount of research suggests Black and Hispanic populations may have lower incidence of FTD relative to White and Asian populations
Lewy body dementia	• Appears to be more common in men, but there have been inconsistent findings in pathologically confirmed studies • Concomitant Alzheimer's pathology is more common in women • Men may show faster rates of cognitive decline than women	• The prevalence of LBD may be lower among Asian populations • Concomitant AD pathology may be more common among Hispanic and Black populations

Abbreviations: AD, Alzheimer's disease; FTD, frontotemporal dementia; LBD, Lewy body dementia.

fewer behavioral changes or potentially because of differences in environmental factors, such as a history of head injury.[68]

There are known challenges in the accurate clinical diagnosis of LBD[69] and this may be especially true for women. Among pathologically confirmed LBD cases, women are less likely to be clinically diagnosed with LBD compared with men and are more likely to be diagnosed with AD due to higher rates of concomitant pathology among women.[70] Other research suggests that the prevalence of LBD among men and women may change depending on the age group. For example, women with LBD may present at an older age and may be more common in men under the age of 75.[70] Several studies using samples from specialty clinics indicate the prevalence of LBD is higher in men compared with women; however, this has not been consistently shown, particularly in community-based samples.[71,72] Data from a large study from nine old age psychiatry/memory clinics in the UK revealed the prevalence of LBD was significantly higher in men compared with women. Men with Parkinson's disease may experience a faster rate of cognitive decline than women.[73–76] Estrogen may serve a protective role in synuclienopathies,[58] even among women who receive estrogen replacement therapy post-menopause.[77]

THE ROLE OF RACE AND ETHNICITY IN DEMENTIA OCCURRENCE AND OUTCOMES

Table 1 summarizes race/ethnicity differences in DSDs. There is a strong body of literature to suggest there are significant differences in the prevalence of DSDs, disease severity at diagnosis, and survival time among racially and ethnically diverse populations.[78–82] However, most clinical studies on neurodegenerative diseases significantly lack substantial representation from diverse populations.[83–85] In fact, a systematic review published in 2021 revealed that 94.7% of the participants pooled across 101 AD studies were White.[83]

A recent study from the United States indicates men and individuals identifying as American Indian and Alaska Native, Black, and Hispanic had a significantly higher prevalence case of DSDs with modifiable risk factors including, smoking, diabetes, physical inactivity, depression, low educational attainment, diabetes, midlife obesity, and midlife HTN, relative to women and individuals identifying as Asian or Non-Hispanic White.[86] Black and Non-Hispanic White individuals have higher rates of APOE e4 alleles compared with Hispanic individuals. APOE e4 carriers from all three groups showed faster declines in memory relative to noncarriers, but there may be group differences in terms of the strength of the relationship between allele status and cognitive impairment.[87]

A large body of evidence suggests that the prevalence of VaD differs by racial and ethnic groups. Neuropathological studies have largely shown that the cerebrovascular disease burden is higher in Black and Hispanic individuals relative to Non-Hispanic White individuals. Older adults in Asia frequently experience HTN and intracranial atherosclerotic disease and may have an increased risk of VaD relative to Non-Hispanic White individuals in Western countries.[88] Studies of Japanese-American and Native Hawaiian patients also reveal high rates of cerebrovascular pathology in this population.[61,89] Researchers have revealed high rates of undiagnosed mild cognitive impairment (MCI) and dementia among older American Indian patients with vascular risk factors relative to other populations.[90] Culturally specific interventions aimed at reducing cardiovascular disease and diabetes are particularly important in reducing vascular-related cognitive impairment in these populations.

Relative to other dementia subtypes, there is a paucity of information regarding racial and ethnic differences in FTD. A previous study examining the prevalence of

DSDs subtypes among diverse older adults found similar rates of FTD in Non-Hispanic White, as well as Asian and Pacific Islander populations and lower prevalence among Black and Hispanic populations.[91]

Similarly, there is limited research on diverse patients with LBD and PDD.[92] LBD may be more common among Non-Hispanic White individuals than other racial or ethnic groups.[91] A recent paper examined clinical features among LBD participants identifying as Black Hispanic, or Non-Hispanic White in the National Alzheimer's Coordinating Center Dataset. It should be noted that 87.6% of the sample identified as Non-Hispanic White. Although there were no significant differences between groups in terms of age at initial presentation or functional abilities, Black and Hispanic participants were more likely to be female, single, and have more cardiovascular risk factors than Non-Hispanic White participants. Hispanic participants reported more severe symptoms of depression relative to the other groups. The prevalence of LBD may be lower among Japanese American and Native Hawaiian populations, but mixed Lewy pathology may be more common among Hispanic and Black populations.[61] One study found higher rates of concomitant AD/Lewy body pathology among Black individuals relative to Non-Hispanic White individuals.

In summary, further studies are needed and it is critical to include individuals from diverse racial and ethnic groups in clinical research, particularly as the field seeks to identify biomarkers with adequate sensitivity and specificity.[93,94]

CLINICS CARE POINTS

- Dementia spectrum disorders affect a large number of older adults worldwide with major impacts on developing countries, women, and minorities.
- Cardiovascular risk factors, lifestyle patterns, comorbidities, and anticholinergic burden are all associated with future risk of dementia spectrum disorders.
- Primary prevention is the key strategy to reduce the burden of dementia spectrum disorders in the absence of disease-modifying treatments.

DISCLOSURE

The authors report no disclosures relevant to the manuscript.

REFERENCES

1. Wilson H, Pagano G, Politis M. Dementia spectrum disorders: lessons learnt from decades with PET research. J Neural Transm (Vienna) 2019;126(3):233–51.
2. Available at: https://www.who.int/news-room/fact-sheets/detail/dementia. Accessed January 20, 2022.
3. Kumar A, Sidhu J, Goyal A, et al. Alzheimer disease. Treasure Island (FL): StatPearls; 2022.
4. Chui HC, Ramirez-Gomez L. Clinical and imaging features of mixed Alzheimer and vascular pathologies. Alzheimers Res Ther 2015;7(1):21.
5. Rahimi J, Kovacs GG. Prevalence of mixed pathologies in the aging brain. Alzheimers Res Ther 2014;6(9):82.
6. Cao Q, Tan CC, Xu W, et al. The prevalence of dementia: a systematic review and meta-analysis. J Alzheimers Dis 2020;73(3):1157–66.
7. Elahi FM, Miller BL. A clinicopathological approach to the diagnosis of dementia. Nat Rev Neurol 2017;13(8):457–76.

8. Brayne C, Miller B. Dementia and aging populations-A global priority for contextualized research and health policy. Plos Med 2017;14(3):e1002275.
9. Collaborators GBDDF. Estimation of the global prevalence of dementia in 2019 and forecasted prevalence in 2050: an analysis for the Global Burden of Disease Study 2019. Lancet Public Health 2022;7(2):e105–25.
10. Collaborators GBDD. Global, regional, and national burden of Alzheimer's disease and other dementias, 1990-2016: a systematic analysis for the Global Burden of Disease Study 2016. Lancet Neurol 2019;18(1):88–106.
11. Knopman DS. The Enigma of decreasing dementia incidence. JAMA Netw Open 2020;3(7):e2011199.
12. Available at: https://www.who.int/news/item/02-09-2021-world-failing-to-address-dementia-challenge. Accessed January 24, 2022.
13. Langa KM, Chernew ME, Kabeto MU, et al. National estimates of the quantity and cost of informal caregiving for the elderly with dementia. J Gen Intern Med 2001; 16(11):770–8.
14. Prince M, Acosta D, Albanese E, et al. Ageing and dementia in low and middle income countries-Using research to engage with public and policy makers. Int Rev Psychiatry 2008;20(4):332–43.
15. The Lancet Healthy L. Care for ageing populations globally. Lancet Healthy Longev 2021;2(4):e180.
16. Islam SM, Purnat TD, Phuong NT, et al. Non-communicable diseases (NCDs) in developing countries: a symposium report. Glob Health 2014;10:81.
17. Pase MP, Satizabal CL, Seshadri S. Role of improved vascular health in the declining incidence of dementia. Stroke 2017;48(7):2013–20.
18. Sousa RM, Ferri CP, Acosta D, et al. The contribution of chronic diseases to the prevalence of dependence among older people in Latin America, China and India: a 10/66 Dementia Research Group population-based survey. BMC Geriatr 2010;10:53.
19. Maestre GE. Assessing dementia in resource-poor regions. Curr Neurol Neurosci Rep 2012;12(5):511–9.
20. Perneczky R. Dementia prevention and reserve against neurodegenerative disease. Dialogues Clin Neurosci 2019;21(1):53–60.
21. Sabayan B, Sorond F. Reducing risk of dementia in older age. JAMA 2017; 317(19):2028.
22. Hughes TF, Ganguli M. Modifiable midlife risk factors for Late-life cognitive impairment and dementia. Curr Psychiatry Rev 2009;5(2):73–92.
23. Zissimopoulos J, Crimmins E, St Clair P. The Value of delaying Alzheimer's disease onset. Forum Health Econ Policy 2014;18(1):25–39.
24. Livingston G, Huntley J, Sommerlad A, et al. Dementia prevention, intervention, and care: 2020 report of the Lancet Commission. Lancet 2020;396(10248): 413–46.
25. Caamano-Isorna F, Corral M, Montes-Martinez A, et al. Education and dementia: a meta-analytic study. Neuroepidemiology 2006;26(4):226–32.
26. Ngandu T, von Strauss E, Helkala EL, et al. Education and dementia: what lies behind the association? Neurology 2007;69(14):1442–50.
27. Xu W, Tan L, Wang HF, et al. Education and risk of dementia: dose-response meta-analysis of prospective cohort studies. Mol Neurobiol 2016;53(5):3113–23.
28. Gudala K, Bansal D, Schifano F, et al. Diabetes mellitus and risk of dementia: a meta-analysis of prospective observational studies. J Diabetes Investig 2013; 4(6):640–50.

29. Zilliox LA, Chadrasekaran K, Kwan JY, et al. Diabetes and cognitive impairment. Curr Diab Rep 2016;16(9):87.
30. Awad N, Gagnon M, Messier C. The relationship between impaired glucose tolerance, type 2 diabetes, and cognitive function. J Clin Exp Neuropsychol 2004; 26(8):1044–80.
31. Qiu C, Winblad B, Fratiglioni L. The age-dependent relation of blood pressure to cognitive function and dementia. Lancet Neurol 2005;4(8):487–99.
32. Sabayan B, Westendorp RG. Blood pressure control and cognitive impairment—why low is not always better. JAMA Intern Med 2015;175(4):586–7.
33. Sabayan B, Wijsman LW, Foster-Dingley JC, et al. Association of visit-to-visit variability in blood pressure with cognitive function in old age: prospective cohort study. BMJ 2013;347:f4600.
34. Stewart R, Xue QL, Masaki K, et al. Change in blood pressure and incident dementia: a 32-year prospective study. Hypertension 2009;54(2):233–40.
35. Mintzer J, Donovan KA, Kindy AZ, et al. Lifestyle Choices and brain health. Front Med (Lausanne) 2019;6:204.
36. Groot C, Hooghiemstra AM, Raijmakers PG, et al. The effect of physical activity on cognitive function in patients with dementia: a meta-analysis of randomized control trials. Ageing Res Rev 2016;25:13–23.
37. Mandolesi L, Polverino A, Montuori S, et al. Effects of physical Exercise on cognitive functioning and Wellbeing: biological and Psychological Benefits. Front Psychol 2018;9:509.
38. Shi L, Chen SJ, Ma MY, et al. Sleep disturbances increase the risk of dementia: a systematic review and meta-analysis. Sleep Med Rev 2018;40:4–16.
39. Xie L, Kang H, Xu Q, et al. Sleep drives metabolite clearance from the adult brain. Science 2013;342(6156):373–7.
40. Zhong G, Wang Y, Zhang Y, et al. Smoking is associated with an increased risk of dementia: a meta-analysis of prospective cohort studies with investigation of potential effect modifiers. PLoS One 2015;10(3):e0118333.
41. Rusanen M, Kivipelto M, Quesenberry CP Jr, et al. Heavy smoking in midlife and long-term risk of Alzheimer disease and vascular dementia. Arch Intern Med 2011;171(4):333–9.
42. Rehm J, Hasan OSM, Black SE, et al. Alcohol use and dementia: a systematic scoping review. Alzheimers Res Ther 2019;11(1):1.
43. van de Rest O, Berendsen AA, Haveman-Nies A, et al. Dietary patterns, cognitive decline, and dementia: a systematic review. Adv Nutr 2015;6(2):154–68.
44. van den Brink AC, Brouwer-Brolsma EM, Berendsen AAM, et al. The Mediterranean, dietary approaches to Stop hypertension (DASH), and Mediterranean-DASH intervention for neurodegenerative delay (MIND) diets are associated with less cognitive decline and a lower risk of Alzheimer's disease-A review. Adv Nutr 2019;10(6):1040–65.
45. Krueger KR, Wilson RS, Kamenetsky JM, et al. Social engagement and cognitive function in old age. Exp Aging Res 2009;35(1):45–60.
46. Lavrencic LM, Richardson C, Harrison SL, et al. Is there a link between cognitive reserve and cognitive function in the Oldest-old? J Gerontol A Biol Sci Med Sci 2018;73(4):499–505.
47. Gardner RC, Burke JF, Nettiksimmons J, et al. Dementia risk after traumatic brain injury vs nonbrain trauma: the role of age and severity. JAMA Neurol 2014;71(12): 1490–7.
48. Gardner RC, Yaffe K. Traumatic brain injury may increase risk of young onset dementia. Ann Neurol 2014;75(3):339–41.

49. Omalu B, Bailes J, Hamilton RL, et al. Emerging histomorphologic phenotypes of chronic traumatic encephalopathy in American athletes. Neurosurgery 2011; 69(1):173–83 [discussion: 183].

50. Fann JR, Ribe AR, Pedersen HS, et al. Long-term risk of dementia among people with traumatic brain injury in Denmark: a population-based observational cohort study. Lancet Psychiatry 2018;5(5):424–31.

51. da Silva J, Goncalves-Pereira M, Xavier M, et al. Affective disorders and risk of developing dementia: systematic review. Br J Psychiatry 2013;202(3):177–86.

52. Wolters FJ, Segufa RA, Darweesh SKL, et al. Coronary heart disease, heart failure, and the risk of dementia: a systematic review and meta-analysis. Alzheimers Dement 2018;14(11):1493–504.

53. van der Velpen IF, Feleus S, Bertens AS, et al. Hemodynamic and serum cardiac markers and risk of cognitive impairment and dementia. Alzheimers Dement 2017;13(4):441–53.

54. Richardson K, Fox C, Maidment I, et al. Anticholinergic drugs and risk of dementia: case-control study. BMJ 2018;361:k1315.

55. Gray SL, Anderson ML, Dublin S, et al. Cumulative use of strong anticholinergics and incident dementia: a prospective cohort study. JAMA Intern Med 2015; 175(3):401–7.

56. Eggink E, Moll van Charante EP, van Gool WA, et al. A population Perspective on prevention of dementia. J Clin Med 2019;8(6).

57. Azad NA, Al Bugami M, Loy-English I. Gender differences in dementia risk factors. Gend Med 2007;4(2):120–9.

58. Ullah MF, Ahmad A, Bhat SH, et al. Impact of sex differences and gender specificity on behavioral characteristics and pathophysiology of neurodegenerative disorders. Neurosci Biobehav Rev 2019;102:95–105.

59. Nebel RA, Aggarwal NT, Barnes LL, et al. Understanding the impact of sex and gender in Alzheimer's disease: a call to action. Alzheimers Dement 2018;14(9): 1171–83.

60. Andersen K, Launer LJ, Dewey ME, et al. Gender differences in the incidence of AD and vascular dementia: the EURODEM studies. EURODEM incidence research group. Neurology 1999;53(9):1992–7.

61. Lim U, Wang S, Park SY, et al. Risk of Alzheimer's disease and related dementia by sex and race/ethnicity: the Multiethnic Cohort Study. Alzheimers Dement 2021. https://doi.org/10.1002/alz.12528.

62. Irvine K, Laws KR, Gale TM, et al. Greater cognitive deterioration in women than men with Alzheimer's disease: a meta analysis. J Clin Exp Neuropsychol 2012; 34(9):989–98.

63. Eikelboom WS, Pan M, Ossenkoppele R, et al. Sex differences in neuropsychiatric symptoms in Alzheimer's disease dementia: a meta-analysis. Alzheimers Res Ther 2022;14(1):48.

64. Wellons M, Ouyang P, Schreiner PJ, et al. Early menopause predicts future coronary heart disease and stroke: the Multi-Ethnic Study of Atherosclerosis. Menopause 2012;19(10):1081–7.

65. Pengo M, Alberici A, Libri I, et al. Sex influences clinical phenotype in frontotemporal dementia. Neurol Sci 2022. https://doi.org/10.1007/s10072-022-06185-7.

66. Rogalski E, Rademaker A, Weintraub S. Primary progressive aphasia: relationship between gender and severity of language impairment. Cogn Behav Neurol 2007;20(1):38–43.

67. Illán-Gala I, Casaletto KB, Borrego-Écija S, et al. Sex differences in the behavioral variant of frontotemporal dementia: a new window to executive and behavioral reserve. Alzheimers Dement 2021;17(8):1329–41.
68. de Boer SCM, Riedl L, van der Lee SJ, et al. Differences in sex distribution between genetic and sporadic frontotemporal dementia. J Alzheimers Dis 2021; 84(3):1153–61.
69. Nelson PT, Jicha GA, Kryscio RJ, et al. Low sensitivity in clinical diagnoses of dementia with Lewy bodies. J Neurol 2010;257(3):359–66.
70. Bayram E, Coughlin DG, Banks SJ, et al. Sex differences for phenotype in pathologically defined dementia with Lewy bodies. J Neurol Neurosurg Psychiatry 2021;92(7):745–50.
71. Schneider JA, Aggarwal NT, Barnes L, et al. The neuropathology of older persons with and without dementia from community versus clinic cohorts. J Alzheimers Dis 2009;18(3):691–701.
72. Farina E, Baglio F, Caffarra P, et al. Frequency and clinical features of Lewy body dementia in Italian memory clinics. Acta Biomed 2009;80(1):57–64.
73. Reekes TH, Higginson CI, Ledbetter CR, et al. Sex specific cognitive differences in Parkinson disease. NPJ Parkinsons Dis 2020;6:7.
74. Bakeberg MC, Gorecki AM, Kenna JE, et al. Differential effects of sex on longitudinal patterns of cognitive decline in Parkinson's disease. J Neurol 2021;268(5): 1903–12.
75. Cholerton B, Johnson CO, Fish B, et al. Sex differences in progression to mild cognitive impairment and dementia in Parkinson's disease. Parkinsonism Relat Disord 2018;50:29–36.
76. Iwaki H, Blauwendraat C, Leonard HL, et al. Differences in the presentation and progression of Parkinson's disease by sex. Mov Disord 2021;36(1):106–17.
77. Song YJ, Li SR, Li XW, et al. The effect of estrogen replacement therapy on Alzheimer's disease and Parkinson's disease in Postmenopausal women: a meta-analysis. Front Neurosci 2020;14:157.
78. Matthews KA, Xu W, Gaglioti AH, et al. Racial and ethnic estimates of Alzheimer's disease and related dementias in the United States (2015-2060) in adults aged ≥65 years. Alzheimers Dement 2019;15(1):17–24.
79. Tsoy E, Kiekhofer RE, Guterman EL, et al. Assessment of racial/ethnic Disparities in Timeliness and Comprehensiveness of dementia diagnosis in California. JAMA Neurol 2021;78(6):657–65.
80. Chen C, Zissimopoulos JM. Racial and ethnic differences in trends in dementia prevalence and risk factors in the United States. Alzheimers Dement (N Y) 2018;4:510–20.
81. Mayeda ER, Glymour MM, Quesenberry CP, et al. Survival after dementia diagnosis in five racial/ethnic groups. Alzheimers Dement 2017;13(7):761–9.
82. Mehta KM, Yeo GW. Systematic review of dementia prevalence and incidence in United States race/ethnic populations. Alzheimers Dement 2017;13(1):72–83.
83. Franzen S, Smith JE, van den Berg E, et al. Diversity in Alzheimer's disease drug trials: the importance of eligibility criteria. Alzheimers Dement 2022;18(4):810–23.
84. Shaw AR, Perales-Puchalt J, Johnson E, et al. Representation of racial and ethnic minority populations in dementia prevention trials: a systematic review. J Prev Alzheimers Dis 2022;9(1):113–8.
85. Brijnath B, Croy S, Sabates J, et al. Including ethnic minorities in dementia research: Recommendations from a scoping review. Alzheimers Dement (N Y) 2022;8(1):e12222.

86. Nianogo RA, Rosenwohl-Mack A, Yaffe K, et al. Risk factors associated with Alzheimer disease and related dementias by sex and race and ethnicity in the US. JAMA Neurol 2022;79(6):584–91.
87. Chan ML, Meyer OL, Farias ST, et al. APOE effects on late life cognitive Trajectories in diverse racial/ethnic groups. J Int Neuropsychol Soc 2022;1–10.
88. Turana Y, Tengkawan J, Chia YC, et al. Hypertension and dementia: a comprehensive review from the HOPE Asia Network. J Clin Hypertens (Greenwich) 2019;21(8):1091–8.
89. Nguyen ML, Huie EZ, Whitmer RA, et al. Neuropathology studies of dementia in US persons other than non-Hispanic Whites. Free Neuropathol 2022;3.
90. Kirkpatrick AC, Stoner JA, Donna-Ferreira F, et al. High rates of undiagnosed vascular cognitive impairment among American Indian veterans. Geroscience 2019;41(1):69–76.
91. Hou CE, Yaffe K, Pérez-Stable EJ, et al. Frequency of dementia etiologies in four ethnic groups. Dement Geriatr Cogn Disord 2006;22(1):42–7.
92. Kurasz AM, Smith GE, McFarland MG, et al. Ethnoracial differences in Lewy body diseases with cognitive impairment. J Alzheimers Dis 2020;77(1):165–74.
93. Barnes LL. Biomarkers for Alzheimer dementia in diverse racial and ethnic minorities-A public health priority. JAMA Neurol 2019;76(3):251–3.
94. Khan MJ, Desaire H, Lopez OL, et al. Why Inclusion Matters for Alzheimer's disease biomarker Discovery in Plasma. J Alzheimers Dis 2021;79(3):1327–44.

Establishing a Diagnosis of Cognitive Impairment and Dementia

Office- and Bedside-based Screening for Cognitive Impairment and the Dementias

Which Tools to Use, Interpreting the Results, and What Are the Next Steps?

David L. Nyenhuis, PhD[a,b,*], Jaclyn Reckow, PhD[a]

KEYWORDS

- Dementia • Cognitive screen • MMSE • MoCA • Mini-Cog

KEY POINTS

- Detection of early cognitive impairment can prevent safety problems and allow treatment for potentially treatable sources of cognitive impairment.
- Choice of a cognitive screen depends on the evidence base of the test, patient population, time constraints, and clinician familiarity.
- Standardized administration of cognitive screens is an essential base to interpretation and diagnostic accuracy.
- Cognitive screens are influenced by non-neurologic factors (eg, education level, age, psychiatric illness, and sensory deficits), which need to be considered when interpreting scores.

INTRODUCTION

The aging population contains increasing rates of cognitive decline and dementia.[1] Cognitive deficits are associated with a variety of neurologic, medical, and psychological conditions, including degenerative dementing illnesses, and other diseases that may negatively impact brain function (eg, diabetes, some cancers, liver disease, stroke/cerebrovascular disease, cardiac conditions, depression, and anxiety), metabolic conditions, endocrine states, medication side-effects, and delirium/encephalopathies. Some of these conditions are reversible with treatment. Although others do not respond to treatment, correct diagnoses may lead to potential resources and care for

[a] Neuropsychology Section, Hauenstein Neuroscience Center, Mercy Health of West Michigan, 220 Cherry Street SE, Grand Rapids, MI 49503, USA; [b] Department of Psychology, LCC International University, Kretingos g. 36, Klaipeda, Lithuania
* Corresponding author.
E-mail address: nyenhuda@mercyhealth.com

Clin Geriatr Med 39 (2023) 15–25
https://doi.org/10.1016/j.cger.2022.07.002
0749-0690/23/© 2022 Elsevier Inc. All rights reserved.

the patient and their caregivers. Health care providers are often the first source patients look to for guidance with cognitive impairment.

An early question for the provider is whether to screen for cognitive impairment. The answer is clearly affirmative when patients or family members present with cognitive concerns or when the provider observes behavior suggestive of cognitive impairment. It is much less clear whether to screen patients without cognitive concerns or symptoms. Recently, the US Preventive Services Task Force[2] recommended that cognitive screening not be completed with non-symptomatic patients, concluding that, "the current evidence is insufficient to assess the balance of benefits and harms of screening for cognitive impairment in older adults (page 757)." Reasons for the decision included the lack of efficacy of treatments for cognitive impairment, especially for non-demented adults, and the poor positive predictive value of screening instruments when used with nonclinical community samples. The Centers for Medicare and Medicaid Services require investigation of cognitive impairment at the annual wellness visit. Although formal cognitive screening is not required, it is suggested as a possibility. The investigation may also be done by direct observation and considering the concerns of friends and family members. Indeed, much information can be gathered using informal methods, such as by asking patients about current events (weather, sports, local events), inquiring about whether medications are properly and consistently used, and asking family members or friends about the patient's daily function skills (eg, medication management, bill paying, driving) and general cognitive status.

Health care workers may feel uncomfortable discussing cognitive matters with patients, and what does not get asked may go unnoticed. Chodish and colleagues[3] found that physicians were not aware of 40% of their patients with cognitive impairment, most likely because they did not investigate the matter. The lack of investigation of potential cognitive deficits may lead to significant safety concerns (eg, poor medication management, driving difficulties) and undertreatment of potentially treatable sources of cognitive impairment.

ASSESSMENT

An ideal cognitive screen will correctly identify patients with cognitive impairment while not pathologizing normal cognition, and will do so in a brief, time-conscious manner. There are numerous cognitive screens available and there is no one-size-fits-all "best" cognitive screen. Choosing a cognitive screen will depend on the patient population, individual patient characteristics, and clinical judgment. Ease of use, time constraints, and evidence of test accuracy will also influence screening tool selection. The following summary highlights three commonly used standardized cognitive screeners.

The Mini-Mental State Examination

The mini-mental state examination (MMSE) is a 30-point cognitive screen that takes approximately 5 to 10 min to administer.[4] It includes questions of orientation, verbal memory registration and short delayed recall, working memory, language, and visuospatial abilities. A cutoff of 23 points or lower is often used as a dementia proxy. The MMSE was originally developed for detecting dementia in a geriatric population and differentiating dementia from other causes of cognitive decline, such as depression.

The MMSE functions best when used for its intended purpose with older adults suspected of dementia. For detecting the presence of dementia in community and primary care samples, scores less than or equal to 24 produce an .87 sensitivity and .82 specificity.[5] Using an education-corrected cut point significantly improves sensitivity but results in more patients without cognitive impairment being sent for further diagnostic testing.

MMSE is less sensitive to mild cognitive changes, such as those seen in mild cognitive impairment (MCI). Meta-analysis of MMSE detection of MCI versus normal controls indicated scores 27 and below optimized sensitivity and specificity.[6] However, use of higher cutoff scores may result in higher rates of false-positive errors, as MMSE scores can be influenced by other factors (eg, age, education level; see interpretive considerations below).

MMSE content is heavily weighted with orientation and language items and has been criticized for poor sensitivity for executive functioning and visuospatial deficits, which are more common in non-Alzheimer's pathology, such as Parkinson's disease and vascular changes. MMSE has ceiling effects that limit its ability to detect MCI and dementia due to Parkinson's disease.[7] Even with adjusting MMSE scores to higher cut points to improve sensitivity, MMSE is less sensitive than the Montreal Cognitive Assessment (MoCA) in detecting cognitive deficits in recall, executive functioning, abstraction, and sustained attention in patients with transient ischemic attacks and stroke.[8]

Montreal Cognitive Assessment

The MoCA was developed as a screening instrument sensitive to early cognitive declines found in MCI.[9] The MoCA test is 30-point screen and takes approximately 10 to 12 min to administer with items covering eight general domains: visuospatial/executive abilities, naming, memory registration (not scored), attention/working memory, abstraction, memory recall, and orientation. An education correction of one additional point is added for patients with ≤12 years of education. Scores ≤25 indicate cognitive impairment. Although originally developed to detect prodromal Alzheimer's disease, MoCA has been validated in detecting cognitive impairment of various etiologies, (including Parkinson's disease[10]), vascular cognitive impairment,[11] and other medical conditions.

The optimal MoCA cutoff score is often debated due to concerns for high rates of false-positive errors. Numerous studies have developed optimal cutoff scores for specific populations. For example, Waldron-Perrine and Axelrod[12] recommend an optimal cutoff of ≤20 for an urban veteran sample, but a low cutoff would be insensitive in other settings. Meta-analysis revealed that an optimal cutoff of less than 23 optimized diagnostic accuracy.[13] Landsheer[14] examined optimal cutoff scores for detecting cognitive impairment using MoCA and found scores between 22 and 25 were most error-prone for interpretation. Instead of a dichotomous interpretation, using two-threshold points (ie, >25 normal; 22–25 uncertain; <22 is impaired) allows providers to apply a more cautious clinical approach to individuals in the uncertain range and avoid overdiagnosis.

The MoCA and MMSE are both 30-point screens but cannot be used interchangeably. When both the MoCA and MMSE were administered in a sample of poststroke or TIA patients, 58% of participants with normal MMSE scores had impaired MoCA scores.[8] Several studies have created "crossover" tables to convert a score on the MMSE to a score on the MoCA to help clinicians interpret scores [for example,[15]]. In general, MoCA is preferred for detecting subtle cognitive changes of various etiologies but should be interpreted with caution as to avoid over-pathologizing cognitively intact individuals.

Mini-Cog

The Mini-Cog[16] is a brief screen that takes approximately 3 to 5 min to administer. It combines two commonly used tasks—three-word memory and clock drawing—to measure memory and executive functioning. Each section is worth three points for up to six total. The Mini-Cog was originally developed to screen for dementia in non-white and low-education populations and has been further validated in US population-based samples.[16] The advantages of the Mini-Cog are the ease of use, brevity, and fewer effects of social factors on scores (eg, education level). A Cochrane review of Mini-Cog accuracy in the primary care setting found limited sensitivity and specificity values for detecting all-cause dementia (.76 and .73, respectively), which led to the lack of support for its use in primary care.[17] The Mini-Cog diagnostic accuracy may be improved significantly by adding measures of functioning, such as the Functional Activities Questionnaire (FAQ).[18]

Other Cognitive Screens

Other cognitive screens with adequate psychometric properties include the Addenbrooke's Cognitive Examination-Revised (ACE-R),[19] Memory Impairment Screen (MIS),[20] and General Practitioner Assessment of Cognition (GPCOG)[21] (details in **Table 1**). A disadvantage of the ACE-R is an administration time of approximately 16 min as opposed to MIS and GPCOG, which take less than 5 min. Newer cognitive screens are frequently being developed. Generally, the choice of the cognitive screen will be influenced by its evidence base, appropriateness of use in primary care settings, and clinician's preference.

APPROACH
Administration and Interpretation of Cognitive Screens

Test examination
The choice of a particular screening test is not as important as the ability to competently administer, score and interpret the chosen test. Most cognitive screening tests include standardized administration directions. For example, the MoCA includes specific, word-for-word instructions found on the MoCA website (mocatest.org), and a certification program. The instructions need to be closely followed. When tests are not given in a standardized manner, it hinders the reliability and validity of the results. For example, if two examiners complete the MoCA using different directions, inter-rater reliability suffers. Similarly, if an examiner completes a screening test on two separate occasions with a patient without consistent directions, test-retest reliability is harmed. Because there is a direct relationship between test reliability and test validity, when test reliability suffers it directly and negatively impacts test validity. Therefore, examiners are strongly encouraged to read through administration directions and practice with non-patient volunteers before administering tests to patients. In addition, when there are multiple examiners in a single practice, it is important that they communicate with each other about test administration issues to ensure the test is administered to patients in a consistent manner across examiners. Finally, it is important to score screening tests accurately. To ensure accurate and consistent scoring, consider having both a primary test scorer and a separate score checker; scoring the test twice and checking for scoring consistency increases scoring accuracy.

Test interpretation: age and education effects
Screening tests, like all cognitive tests, are related to patient-related variables. For example, Ylikoski and colleagues[22] found significant education and age-related variance with the MMSE in their Finnish community sample; the two demographic variables accounted for 10% of the MMSE score's variance in the sample. Correcting the MMSE score for age and education improved the accuracy of the study's MMSE-based dementia diagnoses.

Table 1
Common cognitive screens, domains assessed, and recommended interpretive cutoffs

Test	Administration Length (min)	Cognitive Domains Assessed	Score Ranges	Interpretation (Cutoff for Impairment)
Mini-Mental State Examination (MMSE)	5–10	Orientation Verbal memory registration Memory recall Working memory Language Visuospatial abilities	0–30	≤ 23
Montreal Cognitive Assessment (MoCA)	10–12	Visuospatial/executive Naming Memory registration (not scored) Attention/working memory Abstraction Memory recall Orientation	0–30	≤ 25
Mini-Cog	3–5	Memory Executive functioning	0–6	< 3
Addenbrooke's Cognitive Examination-Revised (ACE-R)	12–20	Attention/orientation Memory Fluency Language Visuospatial	0–100	≤ 88
Memory Impairment Screen (MIS)	4	Memory – free recall and cued recall	0–8	≤ 4
General Practitioner Assessment of Cognition (GPCOG)	2–5[a]	Time Orientation Executive functioning Information Memory Recall Informant Report Section	Patient: 0–9 Informant: 0–6 Total: 0–15	Patient: < 8[a] Informant: < 5 Total: < 11

[a] A two-stage method is used: patients with scores greater than 8 or less than 5 are considered intact and impaired, respectively, and the informant section is not administered. Patients scoring 5 to 8 have the informant section administered.

Rossetti and colleagues[23] completed a normative study with the MoCA in a sample of ethnically diverse community adults. Mean MoCA total scores ranged from 25.2 in persons younger than age 35, to 21.3 in persons from age 70 to 80. Moreover, the 70- to 80-year-old subjects with less than a high-school education earned a mean MoCA score of 16.1, which is approximately 10 points below the recognized MoCA cut score. Other normative studies have shown significant education and age effects with the MoCA, suggesting that the cut score may be too stringent, leading to incorrect classification of patients as cognitively impaired.[24]

In addition to the length of education, the clinician should examine the quality of their patient's education. Education quality in the United States has been lower for many African-American and Hispanic-Americans, especially for African-American elders who were educated in the Southern United States. This has led to differences in performance on cognitive tests, including performance on cognitive screening tests.[25]

Why is age inversely correlated with cognitive performance on screening tests? One potential reason is normal cognitive aging. As persons age, they commonly show a mild cognitive decline, especially in such areas as attention, executive functions, and episodic memory.[26] The causes of normal cognitive aging are not clear; to date, studies have been largely unsuccessful in showing robust and consistent relationships between age-related brain changes (eg, white matter hyperintensity, diffuse atrophy) and age-related cognitive decline.

A second potential reason for age-related effects on cognitive screening tests may be increased risk for previously undetected degenerative disease in older versus younger community participants. Age is a strong risk factor for dementia. It may be that older persons in a community sample were at greater risk than younger persons in the sample to have non-detected, early Alzheimer's disease or other degenerative dementia.

Reasons for the direct relationship between education length/quality and performance of elderly subjects on cognitive screening tests may include a person's facility with being in an assessment situation, their ability to complete verbally-based instruction, and cognitive reserve. Cognitive reserve is the hypothesized relationship between brain development and cognitive skills. It is thought that longer periods of high-quality education experiences result in the brain's ability to find alternative ways to complete cognitive tasks when faced with neuronal damage.[27] It may be that persons with longer periods of high-quality education have the ability to overcome some of the negative brain effects of aging, such as diffuse brain atrophy. Cognitive reserve may even provide clues as to how some persons carry significant Alzheimer's-related pathology burden and yet remain cognitively healthy.

To summarize, the clinician who is interpreting a cognitive screening test score must take into account the age and education of the patient. Education should be examined in terms of length and quality. The strength of relationships between aging and education and screening test performance are especially apparent on the MoCA but may also be seen to a lesser degree with the MMSE. Mini-Cog scores have shown a less consistent relationship with age and education than either the MoCA or MMSE.

Test interpretation: effects of psychiatric illness

Depression and anxiety symptoms have consistently been shown to exert mild but significant effects on neuropsychological tests, including cognitive screening tests.[28] Other studies (eg,[29]) have shown that patients with mood disturbance performed worse than non-depressed control subjects on neuropsychological tests, especially on measures of memory and executive function. Del Brutto and colleagues,[28] in a sample of rural Ecuadorian elders, showed that persons with self-reported elevated depression earned significantly lower MoCA scores than non-depressed individuals, and similar findings have been shown in samples of subjects with diagnosed "severe mental illness.[30] In an electroconvulsive treatment (ECT) study, Obbels and colleagues,[31] showed improvements in MMSE score that corresponded with improved mood measures during and after ECT treatment in a sample of 159 patients, aged 55 and older.

Clinicians need to be alert to the mild but significant effects that mood disturbance and other psychiatric illnesses may have on cognitive screening test results; scores that are 1 to 2 points below expected cut-offs may have been influenced by psychiatric symptoms/illness. Explaining this to patients who score below the cut score may lower their concern that they have a dementing illness. Clinicians may also assure the patient that they will continue to monitor the patient's cognitive status with periodic rescreening to confirm that they are not experiencing a progressive, degenerative condition. Of course, treatment of the psychiatric condition via medication and/or psychotherapy should also be explored.

Test interpretation: medical illness

It is not surprising that persons with diagnosed neurologic conditions often score below standard cut points on cognitive screening tests, because these scores may directly reflect neurologic damage caused by the disease. These include, for example, patients diagnosed with Parkinson's disease, stroke, epilepsy, migraine, multiple sclerosis, and other conditions. It may be more surprising that mild cognitive deficits on cognitive screening tests are often noted in patients with a variety of non-neurologic health concerns, including persons with diabetes mellitus.[32] Zhao and colleagues[33] found that patients with diabetes and high levels of glycated hemoglobin (HbA1c) were more likely to decline on MMSE scores than patients with lower baseline HbA1c levels. Patients with other medical disorders, such as chronic kidney disease,[34] congestive heart failure, and atrial fibrillation,[35] and chronic obstructive pulmonary disease (COPD;[36]) also show lower scores than persons without medical illness. Persons with chronic pain, such as that which is associated with arthritis and fibromyalgia, may also present with cognitive complaints and can be expected to score mildly below established cut-points on cognitive screening tests.[37]

Why should medically ill patients score lower on cognitive screening tests? One reason is potential neurologic underpinnings to the cognitive deficits associated with the illness (eg, diabetes, fibromyalgia). Also, significant medical illness may include chronic pain/malaise and/or psychiatric symptoms, which in turn may negatively affect cognitive performance. Often, the mild deficits associated with illness are related to inconsistent attention and focus, which interfere with consistent cognitive processing speed and learning. Indeed, the cognitive patterns seen on full neuropsychological examinations in these patient groups often show mild deficits and variability on measures of attention, executive functions, and learning, whereas retention memory deficits (ie, rapid forgetting) are not often seen.

Test interpretation: miscellaneous

Other factors that may result in lower screening test results include:

1. Patients for whom English is not their primary language. Involving an interpreter increases the potential variability in the testing environment (eg, if the interpreter does not speak the same dialect as the patient), which decreases examiner control of the testing environment, reliability, and validity.
2. Patients with illiteracy. Patients who do not know how to read or write perform more poorly on cognitive testing of all types. Part of this is because some screening tests

require basic literacy (eg, spelling the word, "WORLD" backward and writing a sentence on the MMSE). Perhaps surprisingly, Illiterate patients perform more poorly on both verbal and nonverbal cognitive tests.[38]

3. Patients with sensory deficits. Patients who are hard of hearing or vision impaired often perform poorly on cognitive screening tests. This likely is related to a lack of accurate communication between the examiner and the test taker, but it also may be because standardized test administration is necessarily altered.

4. Patients with inconsistent test engagement or effort. Some patients do not wish to be tested and do not put forth consistent effort during test examination. Other patients may have an incentive to perform poorly. Clinicians need to be alert to the potential that a patient may see it as in their best interest to perform poorly on a screening test.

5. Practice effects. Although most other factors in this section are related to poorer than average test performance, practice effects result in a patient's performance being artificially elevated. To guard against practice effects, consider using multiple forms of a test (eg, both the MoCA and the Mini-Cog have multiple versions and the MMSE allows for alternative words for learning and recall).

SUMMARY
A Proposed Four-Step Clinical Plan for Patients with Cognitive Concerns

Cognitive screening may be part of a more comprehensive plan for assisting patients with cognitive concerns. The first step of the plan is *education*. When patients bring up cognitive concerns, it is important for clinicians to educate them, especially about normal cognitive aging. Patients should be informed that some mild cognitive change is common, especially in the areas of new learning, attention, and memory. Informing them of the likely normality of their concerns can be reassuring. Other areas of education include the potential roles that depression and anxiety, as well as other psychiatric symptoms, may have in cognitive deficits.

The second step in treating patients with cognitive concerns is *screening*. Choose a screening test that you have time to administer and are comfortable with. Learn to interpret screening results, including how factors introduced in the previous section may influence the obtained screening test score. There are, of course, many different screening test options. We chose to review the MMSE, MoCA, and Mini-Cog because of their frequency of use and the availability of psychometric data. When choosing a screening test, consider choosing the MMSE when evaluating an elderly person for the presence of a dementing illness, especially in situations where false-positive errors (stating that there is cognitive impairment when there is none) are more costly than false negative errors (stating that there is not cognitive impairment when cognitive impairment exists). Consider choosing the MoCA in younger patients, especially in patients with adequate years of quality education, and in patients for whom an evaluation of executive functions is important. As mentioned, the MoCA provides greater sensitivity than the MMSE, but at the cost of lower specificity. Finally, in situations where it is not possible to spend the necessary time for the MMSE or MoCA, consider the Mini-Cog to provide a first look at basic cognitive abilities.

The third step in this process is *follow-up*. After you complete the screening test, educate your patient on how they did and whether follow-up tests are indicated. Follow-up tests may include laboratory tests for potentially reversible causes of cognitive decline. If the patient provides permission, follow-up may also include speaking with their spouse or family members to see if they have noted a decline in cognitive or functional abilities. If depression or anxiety symptoms are significant enough to interfere with everyday life, treatment, such as medications and/or psychotherapy, should be discussed with patients. Finally, let your patient know that you may wish to screen them again for cognitive deficits at a future visit to see if there are changes in cognitive abilities over time. Longitudinal cognitive data is an important potential source of information of possible degenerative cognitive conditions.

Finally, the fourth step is a potential *referral*. You may wish to refer the patient to specialists for additional assessment. This may include neurologists or neuropsychologists for a more comprehensive cognitive and functional assessment. Other specialists may also be able to assist, depending on the results found in your cognitive assessment, and the questions they may raise.

The overall goal for assessment and treatment of your patient's cognitive concerns it to improve your and your patient's understanding of their cognitive condition and to provide assistance with potential treatment and resources. Cognitive screening tests have an important role in this process, and when used properly, greatly improve the care of patients with cognitive concerns.

CLINICS CARE POINTS

- Each cognitive screening test has strengths and weaknesses, and the clinician should choose the test that works best in their clinic
- Cognitive screening tests need to be administered and scored in a standardized manner to not detract from their reliability and validity
- Age, education (length and quality), psychiatric illness, medical illness, effort, illiteracy, and sensory deficits may have significant effects on patients' performance on cognitive screening tests
- Cognitive screening should occur along with education, follow-up, and targeted referrals for effective care of patients with cognitive concerns

DISCLOSURE

Neither Dr D.L. Nyenhuis nor Dr J. Reckow has real or potential conflicts of interest to disclose that pertain to the content of this article.

REFERENCES

1. Plassman BL, Langa KM, Fisher GG, et al. Prevalence of dementia in the United States: the aging, demographics, and memory study. Neuroepidemiology 2007; 29(1–2):125–32.
2. US Preventive Services Task Force, Owens DK, Davidson KW, et al. Screening for cognitive impairment in older adults: US preventive Services task Force recommendation statement. JAMA 2020;323(8):757–63.
3. Chodosh J, Petitti DB, Elliott M, et al. Physician recognition of cognitive impairment: evaluating the need for improvement. J Am Geriatr Soc 2004;52(7):1051–9.
4. Folstein MF, Folstein SE, McHugh PR. Mini-mental state". A practical method for grading the cognitive state of patients for the clinician. J Psychiatr Res 1975; 12(3):189–98.
5. Creavin ST, Wisniewski S, Noel-Storr AH, et al. Mini-Mental State Examination (MMSE) for the detection of dementia in clinically unevaluated people aged 65

and over in community and primary care populations. Cochrane Database Syst Rev 2016;2016(1):CD011145.

6. Ciesielska N, Sokołowski R, Mazur E, et al. Is the Montreal Cognitive Assessment (MoCA) test better suited than the Mini-Mental State Examination (MMSE) in mild cognitive impairment (MCI) detection among people aged over 60? Meta-analysis. Psychiatr Pol 2016;50(5):1039–52.

7. Hoops S, Nazem S, Siderowf AD, et al. Validity of the MoCA and MMSE in the detection of MCI and dementia in Parkinson disease. Neurology 2009;73(21): 1738–45.

8. Pendlebury ST, Cuthbertson FC, Welch SJ, et al. Underestimation of cognitive impairment by Mini-Mental State Examination versus the Montreal Cognitive Assessment in patients with transient ischemic attack and stroke: a population-based study. Stroke 2010;41(6):1290–3.

9. Nasreddine ZS, Phillips NA, Bédirian V, et al. The Montreal Cognitive Assessment, MoCA: a brief screening tool for mild cognitive impairment. J Am Geriatr Soc 2005;53(4):695–9 [published correction appears in J Am Geriatr Soc. 2019 Sep;67(9):1991].

10. Mazancova AF, Růžička E, Jech R, et al. Test the best: classification accuracies of four cognitive rating scales for Parkinson's disease mild cognitive impairment [published online ahead of print, 2020 Jul 17]. Arch Clin Neuropsychol 2020;acaa039. https://doi.org/10.1093/arclin/acaa039.

11. Ghafar MZAA, Miptah HN, O'Caoimh R. Cognitive screening instruments to identify vascular cognitive impairment: a systematic review. Int J Geriatr Psychiatry 2019;34(8):1114–27.

12. Waldron-Perrine B, Axelrod BN. Determining an appropriate cutting score for indication of impairment on the Montreal Cognitive Assessment. Int J Geriatr Psychiatry 2012;27(11):1189–94.

13. Carson N, Leach L, Murphy KJ. A re-examination of Montreal cognitive assessment (MoCA) cutoff scores. Int J Geriatr Psychiatry 2018;33(2):379–88.

14. Landsheer JA. Impact of the Prevalence of cognitive impairment on the accuracy of the Montreal cognitive assessment: the advantage of using two MoCA thresholds to identify error-prone test scores. Alzheimer Dis Assoc Disord 2020;34(3): 248–53.

15. Bergeron D, Flynn K, Verret L, et al. Multicenter validation of an MMSE-MoCA Conversion table. J Am Geriatr Soc 2017;65(5):1067–72.

16. Borson S, Scanlan JM, Chen P, et al. The Mini-Cog as a screen for dementia: validation in a population-based sample. J Am Geriatr Soc 2003;51(10):1451–4.

17. Seitz DP, Chan CC, Newton HT, et al. Mini-Cog for the diagnosis of Alzheimer's disease dementia and other dementias within a primary care setting. Cochrane Database Syst Rev 2018;2(2):CD011415.

18. Steenland NK, Auman CM, Patel PM, et al. Development of a rapid screening instrument for mild cognitive impairment and undiagnosed dementia. J Alzheimers Dis 2008;15(3):419–27.

19. Mioshi E, Dawson K, Mitchell J, et al. The Addenbrooke's Cognitive Examination Revised (ACE-R): a brief cognitive test battery for dementia screening. Int J Geriatr Psychiatry 2006;21(11):1078–85.

20. Buschke H, Kuslansky G, Katz M, et al. Screening for dementia with the memory impairment screen. Neurology 1999;52(2):231–8.

21. Brodaty H, Pond D, Kemp NM, et al. The GPCOG: a new screening test for dementia designed for general practice. J Am Geriatr Soc 2002;50(3):530–4.

22. Ylikoski R, Erkinjuntti T, Sulkava R, et al. Correction for age, education and other demographic variables in the use of the Mini Mental State Examination in Finland. Acta Neurol Scand 1992;85(6):391–6.
23. Rossetti HC, Lacritz LH, Cullum CM, et al. Normative data for the Montreal cognitive assessment (MoCA) in a population-based sample. Neurology 2011;77(13): 1272–5.
24. Malek-Ahmadi M, Powell JJ, Belden CM, et al. Age- and education-adjusted normative data for the Montreal Cognitive Assessment (MoCA) in older adults age 70-99. Neuropsychol Dev Cogn B Aging Neuropsychol Cogn 2015;22(6): 755–61.
25. Mantri S, Nwadiogbu C, Fitts W, et al. Quality of education impacts late-life cognition. Int J Geriatr Psychiatry 2019;34:855–62.
26. Harada CN, Natelson Love MC, Triebel KL. Normal cognitive aging. Clin Geriatr Med 2013;29(4):737–52.
27. Stern Y. Cognitive reserve in ageing and Alzheimer's disease. Lancet Neurol 2012;11(11):1006–12.
28. Del Brutto OH, Mera RM, Del Brutto VJ, et al. Influence of depression, anxiety and stress on cognitive performance in community-dwelling older adults living in rural Ecuador: results of the Atahualpa Project. Geriatr Gerontol Int 2015;15(4):508–14.
29. Lin K, Xu G, Lu W, et al. Neuropsychological performance in melancholic, atypical and undifferentiated major depression during depressed and remitted states: a prospective longitudinal study. J Affect Disord 2014;168:184–91.
30. Musso MW, Cohen AS, Auster TL, et al. Investigation of the Montreal Cognitive Assessment (MoCA) as a cognitive screener in severe mental illness. Psychiatry Res 2014;220(1–2):664–8.
31. Obbels J, Vansteelandt K, Verwijk E, et al. MMSE changes during and after ECT in late-life depression: a prospective study. Am J Geriatr Psychiatry 2019;27(9): 934–44.
32. Dybjer E, Nilsson PM, Engström G, et al. Pre-diabetes and diabetes are independently associated with adverse cognitive test results: a cross-sectional, population-based study. BMC Endocr Disord 2018;18(1):91.
33. Zhao L, Han C, Zheng Z, et al. Risk of mini-mental state examination (MMSE) decline in the elderly with type 2 diabetes: a Chinese community-based cohort study. BMC Endocr Disord 2020;20(1):129.
34. Aggarwal HK, Jain D, Bhavikatti A. Cognitive Dysfunction in patients with chronic kidney disease. Saudi J Kidney Dis Transpl 2020;31(4):796–804.
35. Potter EL, Ramkumar S, Wright L, et al. Associations of subclinical heart failure and atrial fibrillation with mild cognitive impairment: a cross-sectional study in a subclinical heart failure screening programme. BMJ Open 2021;11(7):e045896.
36. Pierobon A, Ranzini L, Torlaschi V, et al. Screening for neuropsychological impairment in COPD patients undergoing rehabilitation. PLoS One 2018;13(8): e0199736.
37. Bair MJ, Krebs EE. Fibromyalgia *Ann Intern Med* 2020;172(5):ITC33–48.
38. Nielsen TR, Jørgensen K. Visuoconstructional abilities in cognitively healthy illiterate Turkish immigrants: a quantitative and qualitative investigation. Clin Neuropsychol 2013;27(4):681–92.

Formal Neuropsychological Testing

Test Batteries, Interpretation, and Added Value in Practice

Victor A. Del Bene, PhD[a,b], Adam Gerstenecker, PhD[a,b],
Ronald M. Lazar, PhD[a,b,c],*

KEYWORDS

- Neuropsychology • Cognition • Cognitive impairment • Dementia

KEY POINTS

- Neuropsychological assessment is a validated, established method to evaluate cognitive and functional decline that is associated with focal neurologic diseases such as stroke and neoplastic disease and can aid in the diagnosis of mild cognitive impairment and dementia from neurodegenerative disease, and cognitive impairment due to other medical conditions (human immunodeficiency virus, congestive heart failure, end-stage renal disease).
- Differential diagnosis and treatment planning of Alzheimer's disease, frontotemporal dementia, vascular dementia, and Lewy body dementia, along with presurgical planning for deep brain stimulation, normal pressure hydrocephalus, solid organ transplantation, and coronary artery bypass grafting are improved with neuropsychological assessment.
- Neuropsychologists are well-positioned to assist patients and their families in understanding their cognitive symptoms and planning for the future, as well as predict disease progression, functional decline, hospitalization, and mortality.

BACKGROUND

In the United States, it is common for neurologists, psychiatrists, and primary care physicians to refer patients for a neuropsychological assessment because of concern of cognitive decline.[1] Clinical neuropsychology, a specialty of clinical psychology, evaluates brain–behavior relationships through performance on standardized

a Department of Neurology, Division of Neuropsychology, University of Alabama at Birmingham Heersink School of Medicine, Birmingham, AL 35294, USA; b The Evelyn F. McKnight Brain Institute, University of Alabama at Birmingham Heersink School of Medicine, Birmingham, AL 35294, USA; c Department of Neurobiology, University of Alabama at Birmingham Heersink School of Medicine, Birmingham, AL 35294, USA
* Corresponding author. Department of Neurology, The UAB Evelyn F. McKnight Brain Institute, University of Alabama at Birmingham, Birmingham, AL 35233.
E-mail address: rlazar@uabmc.edu

Clin Geriatr Med 39 (2023) 27–43
https://doi.org/10.1016/j.cger.2022.07.003
0749-0690/23/© 2022 Elsevier Inc. All rights reserved.

geriatric.theclinics.com

cognitive tests.[2,3] The field has a rich history of research and clinical observation validating the assessment methodology,[4] which has also benefited from the development of neuroimaging.[5] A primary goal of this article is to increase health care providers understanding of neuropsychology and the neuropsychologist's role in improving patient care. When evaluating patients referred for mild cognitive impairment (MCI) or dementia, the purpose of the neuropsychological assessment is to (1) obtain evidence of cognitive and functional decline, (2) determine the presence and severity of a cognitive syndrome, (3) offer a differential diagnosis of the underlying cause (eg, Alzheimer's disease, Lewy body dementia, stroke, end-stage renal disease, depression), and (4) inform treatment planning and recommendations.

There are several core components included in neuropsychological assessment. First, the neuropsychologist conducts a thorough review of all medical records including clinic evaluations, medications, imaging studies, laboratory workup and biomarkers, and other pertinent records. This information is used to guide the clinical interview, test selection, and differential diagnosis considerations. During the interview, the neuropsychologist gathers information about the onset and course of cognitive symptoms, along with physical symptoms, changes in functional status, and emotional symptoms. In addition, gathering details about medical, psychiatric, substance use, and developmental histories, along with demographic factors, family history, and social history (work, education, family life, etc.) is necessary.[6]

Cognitive Test Selection and Interpretation

Cognitive screening is a useful tool in neurology, geriatric, and primary care clinics for the objective detection of cognitive symptoms. As cognitive screening is discussed elsewhere in this issue this topic will not be discussed in detail here, but it is necessary to mention briefly the difference between cognitive screening and a comprehensive neuropsychological assessment.[7,8] Cognitive screening (eg, mini-mental state examination, Montreal Cognitive Assessment [MoCA]) is a useful method to identify in a brief period of time a potential cognitive disorder, but these measures lack the sensitivity and specificity of a comprehensive neuropsychological assessment.[7,9,10] When a patient obtains a low score on a cognitive screener, it is recommended they are referred to a neuropsychologist for a more detailed analysis. Even if an individual with subjective cognitive concerns scores 30/30 on the MoCA, it is still worthwhile to refer them to a neuropsychologist because the cognitive screener may not be sufficiently sensitive to detect cognitive decline in an otherwise high functioning individual,[11–13] particularly in the early, mild stages of a neuropathologic process.

After the clinical interview, the neuropsychologist selects the test battery, which may also include a cognitive screener. Test selection requires knowledge of test properties and which test can best answer the referral question. The neuropsychological test battery covers multiple cognitive domains including, processing speed, attention and working memory, language, visuospatial abilities, learning and memory, executive functioning, and sensorimotor functioning. Although a full review of psychometric theory and the psychometric properties of commonly used tests is beyond the scope of this article, a basic overview is helpful. Psychometrics is a set of test characteristics that permit the measurement of human behaviors, abilities, and traits, such as intelligence quotient (IQ), cognition, and personality. This is done through the administration of standardized tests in a controlled setting (eg, a clinic or research laboratory). For a neuropsychological test to have value, the test must measure the cognitive construct, or underlying skill or ability, in a valid manner (ie, construct validity). In other words, a newly designed memory test with high construct validity will correlate with a previously established standard. The test must also be reliable in measurement, yielding similar performances for each administration. If a test has low reliability, then it is not possible to determine if a change in score is due to a disease or condition, environmental distractors, or bias (ie, noise) introduced by the test.

A strength of the neuropsychological assessment is the structured administration of each test, with a standard set of instructions and clearly delineated scoring criteria.[2] There are also normative standards derived from a carefully selected population. This latter property makes possible the comparison of a person's performance relative to other people with similar demographic characteristics, such as age, education, sex, and presumed premorbid level of function, among others.[14,15] The generalizability of findings is limited by the extent to which normative samples do not take these characteristics into consideration. It is up to the clinician to select the tests targeted to the cognitive domains related to the referral question, the most appropriate normative samples, and calibrations. There are many tests that can be administered across the lifespan and some that are age-specific. The particular relevance of age is that some cognitive domains are differentially affected by aging, such as those involving processing speed, whereas others, such as language, are less affected. As seen in **Table 1**, several commonly used test batteries and frequently used neuropsychological tests are described, with these tests selected to fit the scope of this special issue. Mood questionnaires and measures of personality (ie, Geriatric Depression Scale) are also often included to complement the information gathered during the interview. The importance of assessing for, say, depression, is that cognition is affected by factors other than those which are neuropathologic including psychological state. Functional status can also be evaluated through self- and family-report on questionnaires such as the Lawton Instrumental Activities of Daily Living Scale,[16] or through performance on portions of the Neuropsychological Assessment Battery (eg, Bill Pay),[17] the Texas Functional Living Scale,[18] or the Financial Capacity Instrument.[19] Finally, family-report of executive dysfunction (Frontal Systems Behavior Scale)[20] and neuropsychiatric symptoms (Neuropsychiatric Inventory Questionnaire),[21] are also helpful additions when possible, providing the neuropsychologist the opportunity to better characterize everyday functioning and neuropsychiatric symptoms (eg, hallucinations, agitation, depression).

An important difference between an assessment of mental status as part of the physical examination and neuropsychological testing is that brief cognitive screening measures of naming or recollection of three words have discrete outcomes of "normal" or "abnormal." In contrast, neuropsychological testing evaluates higher-order cognitive domains in which function can lie anywhere along a continuum of ability, ranging from severely impaired (<1st %ile) to very superior (>99th %ile). Many psychological constructs generally fit a normal distribution (ie, Gaussian distribution; **Fig. 1**), which is a symmetric, continuous, probability distribution that is the basis for measuring performance on a test relative to the normative population (ie, reference group that is used to derive the distribution of scores).[2,22] To interpret a person's performance on a particular test, his or her raw score (ie, unadjusted performance) is converted to a standardized score (eg, z-score). These scores can be calculated using the person's raw performance score, and both the population mean and standard deviation values for that particular test (a standard deviation is the extent a score deviates from the average and is a measure of variability). Once a standardized score is calculated, the person's score can then be compared with the normal curve to see how far the performance deviates from "average" (z-score of 0, 50th percentile), and their estimated premorbid baseline. Most people fall broadly within ±1 standard deviation (mean z-score = 0, 16th to 84th percentile) (see **Fig. 1**). As scores become more extreme toward the left tail of the distribution, deficits and

Table 1
Commonly used neuropsychological tests and test batteries

Test	Description
Broad Neuropsychological Batteries	
Dementia rating scale-2	• Global measure that can estimate dementia severity • Cutoff scores for dementia (<123 out of 144); age and education corrected standardized scores also available • Attention, Initiation/Perseveration, Construction, Conceptualization, and Memory subscales
Neuropsychological assessment battery	• Battery of cognitive modules (Attention, Language, Memory, Spatial, and Executive Functioning) • Outcome: standardized scores for each subtest and each module
Repeatable battery for the assessment of neuropsychological status	• Brief assessment of five indices (Immediate Memory, Visuospatial/Constructional, Language, Attention, and Delayed Memory) • Outcome: standardized Total Score, as well as standardized scores for each domain Index, and subtest
Processing Speed/Attention/Working Memory	
Trail making test Part A	• Attention, motor speed, and visual scanning • Outcome: completion time and number of errors
Symbol digit modalities test	• Divided attention and working memory, visual scanning, perceptual speed, and motor speed • Outcome: number of correct in 90 s
Digit span	• Basic auditory attention and working memory • Outcome: longest digit spans forwards, backwards, and sequenced
Language	
Boston naming test	• Confrontation naming; presentation of black and white drawings • Earlier test items are common and they become progressively less common toward the end. • Outcome: total correct, number of stimulus and phonemic cues, and number correct with cueing
Verbal fluency	• How quickly a person can generate words to a letter (FAS/CFL) or to a category (animals); 60 s duration per trial • Outcome: total number of words generated
Western aphasia battery	• Language assessment to assess and characterize aphasia • Can identify and classify the following aphasia syndromes: Global, Broca's, Wernicke's, Isolation, Transcortical Motor, Transcortical Sensory, Conduction, and Anomic • Outcome: performance on subtests of fluency, auditory comprehension, repetition and naming, reading, and writing.
Boston diagnostic aphasia examination	• Language assessment to assess and characterize aphasia • Outcomes: total correct on tests of conversation and expository speech, auditory comprehension, oral expression, reading, and writing.

(continued on next page)

Table 1 (*continued*)	
Test	**Description**
Visuospatial	
Judgment of line orientation	• Measure of spatial perception and orientation • Outcome: total number correct
Hooper visual organization test	• Visual integration • Drawing of common objects that are cut into two or more parts, arranged in an illogical manner, and the patient must integrate and name the item • Outcome: total number correct
Rey complex figure test (RCFT)	• Copy of a complex geometric figure. • Visuoperception, planning/organization, problem solving, motor functioning, and episodic memory (see below) • Outcome: total number of details correctly drawn during Copy trial
Clock drawing	• Visuoperception, construction, and executive functioning • Useful in dementia diagnosis and identifying visual neglect or apraxia • There are multiple quantitative and qualitative approaches to scoring
Memory	
Hopkins verbal learning test - revised	• Auditory-verbal encoding, storage, and retrieval; 12-item, semantically related word list • Outcomes: three learning trials, delayed recall, and recognition trial
California verbal learning TEST	• Auditory-verbal encoding, storage, and retrieval; designed to measure quantity and process (semantic clustering, recency/primacy, interference) • Outcomes: A 16-item, semantically related word list with five learning trials, a distractor word list, and both short/long free and cued recall
Logical memory (Wechsler memory scale – IV)	• Encoding, storage, and retrieval of narrative information • Outcomes: immediate and delayed recall, and recognition
RCFT	• Visual-spatial memory; completed after the Copy trial (see above) • Outcomes: Total number of details drawn correctly after an immediate delay and longer delay. Recognition is also tested.
Brief visual motor test – revised	• Visual-spatial memory • Outcomes: Immediate recall of six shapes and their spatial location across three learning trials, delayed recall total score, and recognition
Executive functioning	
Delis–Kaplan executive function system	• A battery of 9 executive functioning tasks; can be administered in full, or as individual tests • Designed to capture mild-to-severe executive dysfunction

(*continued on next page*)

Table 1 (*continued*)	
Test	**Description**
	• Set-shifting, verbal fluency, inhibition, concept formation, planning/sequencing • Outcomes: completion time, number correct, and number of errors
Wisconsin card sorting test	• An ambiguous card-sorting test where the patient has to match on a characteristic of the cards and is only told "correct" or "incorrect" • Novel hypothesis generation, shifting cognitive strategies, and abstraction • Outcomes: categories matched, loss of set, and number of errors
Trail making test – Part B	• Attention, motor speed, and executive control/set-shifting • Outcome: completion time and number of errors
Stroop color-word inhibition test	• Attention and inhibition of an over-learned behavior (reading) • Three trials: word reading, color reading, and interference trial (ie, incongruent word, "Red" is written in green ink and the correct answer is green, not red) • Outcomes: completion time and number of errors
Sensorimotor	
Grooved pegboard	• Hand-eye coordination, fine motor dexterity, and motor speed • Can be used to lateralize motor functioning: stroke, seizure focus, or a unilateral movement disorder • Outcome: completion time for preferred and non-preferred hand, and number of drops
Grip strength	• Hand strength; can be used to lateralize motor functioning • Outcome: Average of two measurements of squeezing the hand dynamometer for both the preferred and non-preferred hand
University of Pennsylvania smell identification test	• Olfactory function, which can be impaired in a number of neurodegenerative and medical conditions • Outcomes: Number correctly identified

impairments can be identified as the probability of observing such a low score by chance alone diminishes. Not all tests are normally distributed though, and this can produce floor or ceiling effects when the tails of the distribution are truncated. This can influence test interpretation and it is imperative that neuropsychologists consider this when interpreting performance on a test with a nonnormal distribution. For example, in patients who are post-carotid artery stenting (CAS), there is evidence that ignoring floor and ceiling effects results in underestimating the benefit of CAS on cognition.[23] When selecting tests and interpreting performance, these factors are considered to ensure an accurate evaluation and interpretation.

When evaluating a patient, neuropsychologists always consider the individual's premorbid level of functioning, as most clinical referrals seek to address whether a change in cognition has occurred. There is some utility to using education and

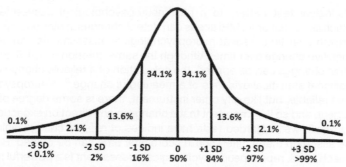

Fig. 1. Example of the normal distribution. *Note.* An example of the normal distribution with demarcations for each standard deviation. As can be seen, most scores fall within 1 standard deviation of the mean (z-score = 0, ±1; equivalent 50th percentile). As scores deviate further from the mean, the probability of their occurrence declines and it is possible to make inferences about cognitive deficits, impairments, and decline.

occupational history as a basis for estimating change. A more empirical approach that minimizes errors in the interpretation of findings, however, is to administer an oral word-reading test that is correlated with Full-Scale IQ[24,25] and is considered a "hold test" because it is relatively resilient to brain injury and most cognitive deficits, other than an expressive language disorder. Clinically, these scores are used as anchors from which inferences of cognitive decline on other neuropsychological tests can be made. This is particularly important for patients whose premorbid functioning is estimated below or above the average range. As an example, consider the following cognitive profiles in two patients in which all test scores are between the 25th and 50th percentiles. Patient A is a high school graduate with a premorbid estimate at the 45th percentile—in this case, all scores are interpreted as unchanged. Conversely, patient B is a physician with a premorbid estimate at the 95th percentile—in this case, these average scores reflect a clinically significant decline for this individual. Despite the comparability of scores for these two individuals, failure to appreciate Patient B's superior premorbid level of functioning would lead to the erroneous conclusion that his or her cognition is intact.

Whether a cognitive screener or neuropsychological test battery is administered, it can be often difficult to determine if a patient is fully engaged and providing effort, which is vital when interpreting the cognitive profile. When evaluating patients of any age, neuropsychologists are mindful of engagement and effort when interpreting test performance to avoid erroneous conclusions. Professional neuropsychology societies call for the use of performance validity tests.[26,27] These measures have been validated for both MCI and mild dementia patient groups, and well traumatic brain injury,[28] epilepsy,[29] other neurologic, neuropsychiatric, and medical conditions.[30] There is always a risk of inferring a failure of effort when there is also true cognitive impairment[31–33] and caution when interpreting low-performance validity scores is warranted.

After the estimate of premorbid functioning is determined and it is likely the patient provided adequate effort, the cognitive profile can be interpreted. Before interpreting cognitive test performance, neuropsychologists set an *a priori* criterion for differentiating impaired from intact scores. A common approach is to use the following cutoffs of 1, 1.5, or 2 standard deviations below a person's presumed baseline to identify cognitive decline.[2,34] Although this approach can detect a cognitive change and is widely used, a more sensitive method is to compare current performance on a neuropsychological test battery to a past neuropsychological assessment, when possible. Much like serial brain MRI scans can detect changes in hippocampal atrophy or tumor growth over time, repeat neuropsychological assessments can be used to evaluate cognitive change over time. Although the same criterion of 1, 1.5, and 2 standard deviation changes can be applied, the calculation of a reliable change index can provide additional statistical evidence of a meaningful change.[35] Neuropsychological measures are reliable, but like any other instrument, there is some degree of variation of measurement, and so it is important that a change in any direction exceeds this variability. As a result, well-regarded tests have indices of reliable change which makes possible the assertion that a difference in score over time can be trusted. Regardless of the approach used, repeat neuropsychological assessment is a powerful method to detect the change and can help improve diagnostic clarity, particularly in the early stages of a neurodegenerative process when there may be greater subjective than objective cognitive change at the baseline assessment.

The pattern of decline is also important. As it is not uncommon for healthy, cognitively intact individuals to produce one or two low scores across a comprehensive neuropsychological test battery,[36] neuropsychologists look for patterns of atypically low scores and if this profile is consistent with neurologic symptoms, clinical history, and neuroimaging. At times, neuropsychological profiles can also be variable without a clear pattern. Elevated levels of intra-individual, or within-person, cognitive variability across the neuropsychological test battery can also be a useful marker of central nervous system dysfunction, with elevated levels of variability observed in those with MCI, mild dementia, and human immunodeficiency virus (HIV)-associated neurocognitive disorder.[37–39]

Once the neuropsychological profile is analyzed and interpreted, the neuropsychologist makes a cognitive diagnosis, such as MCI (eg, mild neurocognitive disorder), or dementia (eg, major neurocognitive disorder). A diagnostic flow chart based on The Diagnostic and Statistical Manual of Mental Disorders, Fifth Edition (DSM-5) criteria for the mild and major neurocognitive disorder is depicted in **Fig. 2**. If a cognitive diagnosis is made, then the neuropsychologist offers a differential diagnosis regarding the underlying cause of the patient's cognitive syndrome. As seen in **Table 2**, common causes of cognitive impairment and dementia include Alzheimer's disease, stroke/vascular cognitive impairment, frontotemporal dementia (behavioral variant, primary progressive aphasia), Lewy body dementia, and Parkinson's disease. Other neurologic causes of dementia include Huntington's disease, normal pressure hydrocephalus, multiple sclerosis, and atypical parkinsonian conditions (multiple systems atrophy, progressive supranuclear palsy, corticobasal degeneration). Medical conditions, such as HIV, congestive heart failure, carotid artery stenosis, chronic kidney disease, obstructive sleep apnea, insomnia, delirium, diabetes, hypothyroidism, cancer, and cancer-related treatments can also lead to cognitive impairment.

When interpreting the neuropsychological profile, neuropsychologists must also consider behavioral observations and approaches to test taking. Demeanor, interpersonal abilities, errors in expressive language, disinhibition, rapid forgetting, sensorimotor deficits, and affective state during the assessment all provide contextual information needed to interpret an impaired performance.[2] For example, in behavioral variant frontotemporal dementia (bvFTD), apathy, diminished empathy, and inappropriate social behaviors, are important clinical signs,[40] with these deficits not commonly captured by psychometric test performance alone. Psychometric test scores, including the quantification of errors (ie, number of commission or omission errors), when paired with behavioral observation (ie, rapid forgetting of instructions, inappropriate behaviors, stimulus-bound behaviors) can further differentiate those

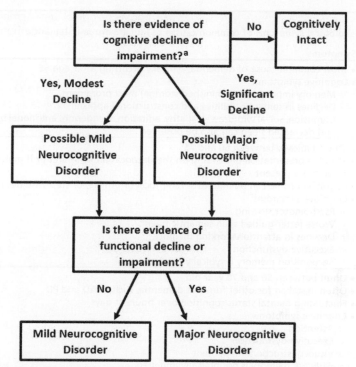

Fig. 2. DSM-5 diagnostic flow chart for mild and major neurocognitive disorder. [a]Not due to delirium or a psychiatric illness.

with Alzheimer's disease dementia and bvFTD.[41,42] The process of how a patient approaches a test is also an important behavioral observation. When considering the response patterns on a word-list memory test (ie, primacy, middle, and recency effects), older adults with major depression recall words from earlier in the list (primacy effect), whereas older adults with Alzheimer's disease recall words from the end of the list (primacy effect).[43] Other behavioral observations can help improve conceptualization and diagnosis, such as motor symptoms (high-frequency tremor on graphomotor tests) or signs of poststroke visual neglect on tests of visual scanning.

After a differential diagnosis is discussed in the neuropsychology report, the neuropsychologist provides specific recommendations to the patient and caregiver. These can include further workup (imaging, blood, cerebrospinal fluid, and genetic biomarkers), referrals to specialists (neurology, geriatrician, and psychiatry), review of medications (polypharmacy, anticholinergic side effects), strategies to reduce vascular risk factors, lifestyle modifications (eg, exercise, diet, sleep, stress reduction, smoking and alcohol reduction, and cessation), recommendations regarding driving, and compensatory strategies. Family recommendations, such as future planning, support groups, respite care, and behavioral management strategies can also be provided by the neuropsychologist. This information is communicated to the referring physician in the neuropsychological report and to the patient during a feedback session.

DISCUSSION

Clinical neuropsychological assessment is a comprehensive, effective method that can identify cognitive and functional decline in the geriatric population. This approach

	Symptoms
Table 2	
Neuropsychological symptoms of common causes of impairment and dementia	
AD	• Most common cause of dementia, typically occurring after age 65 • Cognitive symptoms: ○ Memory impairment (diminished storage) most prominent, ○ Declines in semantic abilities and constructional apraxia. ○ Confusion, social withdrawal, apathy, agitation, wandering, emotional blunting, and decreased sleep can also be observed
VCI	• Onset typically between 60 and 75 • Variable presentation depending on the size/location of infarct or if multiple infarcts are present • Cognitive profile can be mild-to-severe, focal or diffuse, or step-wise decline • Cognitive symptoms: ○ Psychomotor slowing ○ Worse letter-guided than semantic fluency ○ Declines in attention/working memory, ○ Executive dysfunction. ○ Recognition memory is typically preserved
LBD	• Onset between 50 and 70 year old • Often mistaken for other forms of dementia, such as AD and PD • Fluctuating mental status/cognition over hours or days • Cognitive symptoms: ○ Attention ○ Executive dysfunction ○ Visuoconstruction impairment ○ Early on, memory is not typically impaired. ○ Well-formed visual hallucinations are common and often do not cause distress
bvFTD	• Onset typically between 50 and 60 • Behavioral variant of frontal lobar degeneration • Progression often is more rapid than AD • Personality, behavioral, and cognitive changes: ○ Social withdrawal ○ Inappropriate social behaviors and diminished social awareness ○ Apathy and emotional blunting ○ Impulsivity, perseverative behaviors, stimulus-bound behaviors ○ Changes in sexual behaviors ○ Impaired mental flexibility, ○ Poor planning/disorganization ○ Distractibility ○ Deficient problem solving
PPA	• Onset typically between 50 and 60 • Language variant of frontal lobar degeneration • Progression often is more rapid than AD • Language impairment is the first cognitive symptom and the most salient deficit ○ Word-finding deficits ○ Frequent pauses/halting speech ○ Poor grammar ○ Naming impairments ○ Difficulty comprehending written or spoken language, particularly single words ○ Difficulty repeating words, sentences, or phrases ○ Apraxia of speech ○ Dysarthria • Three subtypes include progressive non-fluent aphasia, semantic aphasia, and logopenic aphasia

(continued on next page)

Table 2 (continued)	
	Symptoms

PD	• Onset between 60 and 70
	• Dementia does not invariably develop in all people with PD
	• Unilateral motor symptoms develop before cognitive symptoms
	• Apathy, depression, and anxiety are common
	• Cognitive symptoms
	   ○ Executive dysfunction
	   ○ Memory declines with intact recognition
	   ○ Bradyphrenia/slowing
	   ○ Impaired visuospatial abilities

CHF	• Affects 1%–2% of the adult population; 6%–10% in people over age 65
	• Cognitive impairment can interfere with self-care and medical decision making
	• Cognitive impairment correlated with increased mortality and hospital re-admission
	• Cognitive symptoms:
	   ○ Memory decline
	   ○ Inattention & working memory declines
	   ○ Executive dysfunction
	   ○ Psychomotor slowing
	• Heart transplantation can potentially improve cognitive functioning

CKD	• Affects 1 in 10 people; rates projected to increase because of comorbidity
	• Cognitive symptoms for early-stage CKD:
	   ○ Inattention
	   ○ Processing speed slowing
	   ○ Memory retrieval deficits
	• Cognitive symptoms for moderate stage CKD:
	   ○ Executive dysfunction
	   ○ Verbal fluency declines
	   ○ Disorientation/concentration declines
	   ○ Impaired story memory
	• Cognitive symptoms for severe stage CKD
	   ○ Impaired cognitive control
	   ○ Immediate and delayed memory impairment
	   ○ Visuospatial impairment
	• There can be improvements in attention and working memory 1 year post-kidney transplantation

OSA	• Occurs in 3% of normal weight and >20% of obese people
	• Affects men more than women
	• Increases the risk of stroke and dementia
	• Cognitive symptoms:
	   ○ Inattention
	   ○ Slowed psychomotor speed
	   ○ Verbal fluency declines/word-retrieval difficulties
	   ○ Memory retrieval difficulties and diminished encoding
	   ○ Executive dysfunction
	• CPAP can slow the rate of cognitive decline, reduce risk of stroke and dementia, and may help improve cognition depending on severity

HIV	• HIV-associated neurocognitive disorder (HAND) subgroups:
	   ○ Asymptomatic neurocognitive impairment (ANI)
	   ○ Minor neurocognitive disorder (MND)
	   ○ HIV-associated dementia (HAD)
	• HAND can occur in 20% of people living with HIV, including those receiving combination antiretroviral therapy

(continued on next page)

Table 2 (continued)
Symptoms
• Cognitive symptoms: ○ Inattention/concentration difficulties ○ Memory decline ○ Slowed processing speed ○ Word-finding difficulties ○ Difficulty with planning and organization

Symptoms represent reflect earlier disease course before transitioning to a moderate-to-severe dementia syndrome and global cognitive impairment.

Abbreviations: AD, Alzheimer's disease; bvFTD, Behavioral Variant FTD; CHF, congestive heart failure; CKD, chronic kidney disease; FTD, frontotemporal dementia; HIV, Human Immunodeficiency Virus; LBD, lewy body dementia with lewy bodies; OSA, obstructive sleep apnea; PD, Parkinson's disease; PPA, primary progressive aphasia; VCI, vascular cognitive impairment.

to evaluating cognitive status has been empirically validated with regard to domains of function and has been associated with brain physiology and anatomy, disease pathology, and important psychosocial factors. Despite the strengths of neuropsychological assessment, there are limitations.

In the absence of repeat neuropsychological assessment, the clinical neuropsychologist is left with a cross-sectional model examining a person's performance on complex tasks at a single point in time, making it difficult to appreciate subtle declines from baseline. Repeat neuropsychological assessment allows for both direct comparisons to the person's past neuropsychological evaluation, and the normative samples. Test and normative sample selection can also bias interpretation and diagnosis.[44] Memory, language, and executive functioning are all very complex cognitive processes that can be measured with multiple tests, but the standardized procedures and outcomes may not be equivalent across tests (eg, different time delays for memory recall). For example, memory can be evaluated through the rote recall of a word-list or recall of a narrative that provides a cohesive way to organize information. The test paradigms selected provide different information about the person's memory functioning.

A notable criticism of the current state of neuropsychology is that many neuropsychological tests have limited diagnostic accuracy when applied to the performance of non-White individuals, particularly people with limited education, and those from culturally different backgrounds, which raises clinical, ethical, and practical issues.[45–47] Primary language, bilingualism, and level of acculturation must always be considered when selecting tests, working with interpreters, and interpreting scores.[48–51] Ideally, when a patient's primary language is not English, the best practice is to refer the individual to a neuropsychologist fluent in the patient's language who can administer culturally appropriate tests. However, this may not always be possible, and an interpreter will then be needed to complete the evaluation. The use of interpreters has limitations, including the availability of an interpreter for less commonly spoken languages in the United States, different dialects, level of familiarity with cognitive testing, problems with translating the test material between English and another language, and nonrepresentative normative samples. Finally, there are also considerations of race, with research documenting differences in cognitive test performance, rates of dementia diagnosis, and differences in neuropsychiatric symptoms between Black and White individuals.[52–54] However, race is often used as a proxy for other difficult-to-measure markers of disparities, such as education quality, socioeconomic status, racism, discrimination, and stereotyped threat.[45,54–56] Moreover, race-based group differences do not reflect group biological differences, but rather complex historical and psychosocial factors.

Added Value to Clinical Practice

There is ample evidence that neuropsychological assessment improves diagnostic accuracy for MCI and dementia due to Alzheimer's disease, frontotemporal dementia, vascular dementia, and Lewy body dementia[57] (see **Table 2**). Neuropsychological assessment also predicts outcomes for surgical interventions, such as deep brain stimulation in Parkinson's disease, shunt placement for normal pressure hydrocephalus, post-kidney transplant medication adherence, and cognitive outcomes postcoronary artery bypass grafting and CAS.[23,58–61] Moreover, neuropsychological assessment can predict disease progression, functional decline, risk of hospitalization, and mortality,[57,62–67] all of which have profound medical, psychological, and financial implications for the patient, their families, and treatment team. Regarding family caregivers, 20% of caregivers of people with Alzheimer's disease and 40% of caregivers of people with Lewy body dementia reported moderate-to-high caregiver burden, including an increased risk of the caregiver manifesting psychiatric symptoms.[68] A similar pattern of elevated depression and anxiety is observed in caregivers of stroke patients.[69] The neuropsychologist can address the risk and signs of caregiver burden with family members to help support the family system more broadly. Neuropsychology is a value-adding service that is vital for hospital systems and physicians wanting to provide the highest quality of patient care, and as a means for patients and their families to develop an understanding of cognitive symptoms and the expected clinical course.

SUMMARY

Cognition is a highly sensitive marker of central nervous system dysfunction. In the case of cognitive impairment and dementia, cognitive decline can be evaluated by neuropsychologists using validated, empirically supported psychometric tests of cognition. Test performances are interpreted in the context of medical and psychiatric history, psychosocial factors, and behavioral observations. Neuropsychologists are well-positioned to identify cognitive and functional decline, diagnose a cognitive disorder, provide a differential diagnosis for the underlying cause, track symptom progression, and predict future decline, hospitalization, and mortality. The neuropsychologist is also able to provide treatment recommendations for physicians, the patient, and their family, including the need for the family to plan for the future and to manage the caregiver burden.

CLINICS CARE POINTS

- Cognitive screening alone is not sufficient to identify and diagnosis a cognitive disorder for most patients, but a comprehensive neuropsychological assessment is sufficiently sensitive to improve diagnostic clarity and inform treatment planning.

- Neuropsychological assessment can track progression from mild cognitive impairment to dementia, differentiate various underlying neurodegenerative causes for a cognitive disorder (Alzheimer's disease, vascular dementia, Lewy body dementia, frontotemporal dementia), and differentiate a neurodegenerative illness from focal disease, systemic illness, and from a psychiatric illness.

- When possible, repeat neuropsychological assessment provides the most robust evidence for cognitive change over time or following treatment.

- The neuropsychologist considers the premorbid level of function when determining whether a low score is truly a change. Similarly, factors of culture, education, socioeconomic status, primary language, and acculturation are paramount for the neuropsychologist to consider when interpreting test performance and making a diagnosis.

- The neuropsychologist is well-positioned to explain cognitive symptoms to patients and their families, introduce compensatory or behavioral management strategies, and to guide the families toward planning for the future and avoiding caregiver burnout.

DISCLOSURE

No financial conflicts of interest. This article was possible in part by the UAB McKnight Brain Institute.

REFERENCES

1. Sweet JJ, Klipfel KM, Nelson NW, et al. Professional practices, beliefs, and incomes of US neuropsychologists: the AACN, NAN, SCN 2020 practice and "salary survey". Clin Neuropsychologist 2021;35(1):7–80.
2. Lezak MD, Howieson DB, Loring DW, et al. Neuropsychological assessment. USA: Oxford University Press; 2004.
3. Vakil E. Neuropsychological assessment: Principles, rationale, and challenges. J Clin Exp Neuropsychol 2012;34(2):135–50.
4. Barr WB. Historical development of the neuropsychological test battery. Textbook Clin Neuropsychol 2008;3–17.
5. Price CJ. The evolution of cognitive models: from neuropsychology to neuroimaging and back. Cortex 2018;107:37–49.
6. Assuras S, Levin B. Special considerations for the neuropsychological interview with older adults. Handbook on the Neuropsychology of Aging and Dementia. Springer; 2013. p. 3–9.
7. Block CK, Johnson-Greene D, Pliskin N, et al. Discriminating cognitive screening and cognitive testing from neuropsychological assessment: implications for professional practice. Clin Neuropsychologist 2017;31(3):487–500.
8. Roebuck-Spencer TM, Glen T, Puente AE, et al. Cognitive screening tests versus comprehensive neuropsychological test batteries: a national academy of neuropsychology education paper. Arch Clin Neuropsychol 2017;32(4):491–8.
9. Chan E, Khan S, Oliver R, et al. Underestimation of cognitive impairments by the Montreal Cognitive Assessment (MoCA) in an acute stroke unit population. J Neurol Sci 2014;343(1–2):176–9.
10. Moafmashhadi P, Koski L. Limitations for interpreting failure on individual subtests of the Montreal Cognitive Assessment. J Geriatr Psychiatry Neurol 2013;26(1):19–28.
11. Garrett KD, Perry W, Williams B, et al. Cognitive screening tools for late career physicians: a critical review. J Geriatr Psychiatry Neurol 2021;34(3):171–80.
12. Gaudet CE, Del Bene VA. Neuropsychological assessment of the aging physician: a review and commentary. J Geriatr Psychiatry Neurol 2021;35(3):271–9.
13. Del Bene VA, Brandt J. Identifying neuropsychologically impaired physicians. Clin Neuropsychologist 2020;34(2):318–31.
14. Heaton RK, Ryan L, Grant I. Demographic influences and use of demographically corrected norms in neuropsychological assessment. In: Grant I, Adams KM, editors. Neuropsychological Assessment of Neuropsychiatric and Neuromedical Disorders. 3rd ed. New York: Oxford University Press; 2019. p. 127–58.

15. Testa SM, Winicki JM, Pearlson GD, et al. Accounting for estimated IQ in neuro-psychological test performance with regression-based techniques. J Int Neuro-psychol Soc 2009;15(6):1012–22.
16. Graf C. The Lawton instrumental activities of daily living scale. AJN The Am J Nurs 2008;108(4):52–62.
17. Iverson GL, Brooks BL, White T, Stern RA. Neuropsychological Assessment Battery (NAB): Introduction and advanced interpretation. In: Horton Jr AM, Wedding D, editors. The Neuropsychology Handbook. New York: Springer Publishing Inc; 2008. p. 279–343.
18. Cullum CM, Saine K, Chan LD, et al. Performance-based instrument to assess functional capacity in dementia: the Texas Functional Living Scale. Cogn Behav Neurol 2001;14(2):103–8.
19. Gerstenecker A, Eakin A, Triebel K, et al. Age and education corrected older adult normative data for a short form version of the Financial Capacity Instrument. Psychol Assess 2016;28(6):737.
20. Malloy P, Tremont G, Grace J, et al. The Frontal Systems Behavior Scale discriminates frontotemporal dementia from Alzheimer's disease. Alzheimer's Demen 2007;3(3):200–3.
21. Kaufer DI, Cummings JL, Ketchel P, et al. Validation of the NPI-Q, a brief clinical form of the Neuropsychiatric Inventory. J neuropsychiatry Clin neurosciences 2000;12(2):233–9.
22. Strauss E., Sherman, E.M.S., et al., Compendium of neuropsychological tests: administration, norms, and commentary. 3rd ed. Oxford UK: Oxford University Press, 2006.
23. Scherr M, Kunz A, Doll A, et al. Ignoring floor and ceiling effects may underestimate the effect of carotid artery stenting on cognitive performance. J neurointerventional Surg 2016;8(7):747–51.
24. Shura RD, Ord AS, Martindale SL, et al. Test of Premorbid Functioning: you're doing it wrong, but does it matter? Arch Clin Neuropsychol 2022;37(5):1035–40.
25. Mullen CM, Fouty HE. Comparison of the WRAT4 reading subtest and the WTAR for estimating premorbid ability level. Appl Neuropsychol Adult. 2014;21(1):69–72.
26. Sweet JJ, Heilbronner RL, Morgan JE, et al. American Academy of Clinical Neuropsychology (AACN) 2021 consensus statement on validity assessment: Update of the 2009 AACN consensus conference statement on neuropsychological assessment of effort, response bias, and malingering. The Clin Neuropsychologist 2021;35(6):1053–106.
27. Bush SS, Ruff RM, Tröster AI, et al. Symptom validity assessment: practice issues and medical necessity NAN policy & planning committee. Arch Clin Neuropsychol 2005;20(4):419–26.
28. Bigler ED. Effort, symptom validity testing, performance validity testing and traumatic brain injury. Brain Inj 2014;28(13–14):1623–38.
29. Maiman M, Del Bene VA, MacAllister WS, et al. Reliable digit span: does it adequately measure suboptimal effort in an adult epilepsy population? Arch Clin Neuropsychol 2019;34(2):259–67.
30. McWhirter L, Ritchie CW, Stone J, et al. Performance validity test failure in clinical populations—a systematic review. J Neurol Neurosurg Psychiatr 2020;91(9):945–52.
31. Martin PK, Schroeder RW, Olsen DH. Performance validity in the dementia clinic: specificity of validity tests when used individually and in aggregate across levels of cognitive impairment severity. The Clin Neuropsychologist 2022;36(1):165–88.
32. Clark H, Martin P, Schroeder R. Digit span Forward as a performance validity test in dementia evaluations: specificity in mild cognitive impairment, mild dementia, and moderate dementia. Arch Clin Neuropsychol 2019;34(6):837.

33. Corriveau-Lecavalier N, Alden EC, Stricker NH, et al. Failed performance on the test of memory malingering and Misdiagnosis in individuals with early-onset Dysexecutive Alzheimer's disease. Arch Clin Neuropsychol 2022. https://doi.org/10.1093/arclin/acac016.

34. Mitrushina M, Boone KB, Razani J, et al. Handbook of normative data for neuropsychological assessment. Oxford University Press; 2005.

35. Duff K. Evidence-based indicators of neuropsychological change in the individual patient: relevant concepts and methods. Arch Clin Neuropsychol 2012; 27(3):248–61.

36. Binder LM, Iverson GL, Brooks BL. To err is human:"Abnormal" neuropsychological scores and variability are common in healthy adults. Arch Clin Neuropsychol 2009;24(1):31–46.

37. Reckess GZ, Varvaris M, Gordon B, et al. Within-person distributions of neuropsychological test scores as a function of dementia severity. Neuropsychology 2014; 28(2):254.

38. Holtzer R, Verghese J, Wang C, et al. Within-person across-neuropsychological test variability and incident dementia. Jama 2008;300(7):823–30.

39. Vance DE, Del Bene VA, Frank JS, et al. Cognitive intra-individual variability in HIV: an Integrative review. Neuropsychol Rev 2021;1–22.

40. Johnen A, Bertoux M. Psychological and cognitive markers of behavioral variant frontotemporal dementia–A clinical neuropsychologist's view on diagnostic criteria and beyond. Front Neurol 2019;10:594.

41. Hutchinson A, Mathias J. Neuropsychological deficits in frontotemporal dementia and Alzheimer's disease: a meta-analytic review. J Neurol Neurosurg Psychiatry 2007;78(9):917–28.

42. Thompson JC, Stopford CL, Snowden JS, et al. Qualitative neuropsychological performance characteristics in frontotemporal dementia and Alzheimer's disease. J Neurol Neurosurg Psychiatry 2005;76(7):920–7.

43. Foldi NS, Brickman AM, Schaefer LA, et al. Distinct serial position profiles and neuropsychological measures differentiate late life depression from normal aging and Alzheimer's disease. Psychiatry Res 2003;120(1):71–84.

44. Howieson D. Current limitations of neuropsychological tests and assessment procedures. The Clin Neuropsychologist 2019;33(2):200–8.

45. Manly JJ. Critical issues in cultural neuropsychology: Profit from diversity. Neuropsychol Rev 2008;18(3):179–83.

46. Brickman AM, Cabo R, Manly JJ. Ethical issues in cross-cultural neuropsychology. Appl Neuropsychol 2006;13(2):91–100.

47. Pedraza O, Mungas D. Measurement in cross-cultural neuropsychology. Neuropsychol Rev 2008;18(3):184–93.

48. Arce Rentería M, Casalletto K, Tom S, et al. The contributions of active Spanish-English bilingualism to cognitive reserve among older hispanic adults living in California. Arch Clin Neuropsychol 2019;34(7):1235.

49. Tan YW, Burgess GH, Green RJ. The effects of acculturation on neuropsychological test performance: a systematic literature review. The Clin Neuropsychologist 2021;35(3):541–71.

50. Fujii D, Santos O, Della Malva L. Interpreter-assisted neuropsychological assessment: clinical considerations. Understanding cross-cultural neuropsychology: Science, testing and challenges. 2022.

51. Manly JJ, Byrd DA, Touradji P, et al. Acculturation, reading level, and neuropsychological test performance among African American elders. Appl Neuropsychol 2004;11(1):37–46.

52. Lennon JC, Aita SL, Del Bene VA, et al. Black and White individuals differ in dementia prevalence, risk factors, and symptomatic presentation. Alzheimer's & Dementia; 2021.
53. Werry AE, Daniel M, Bergström B. Group differences in normal neuropsychological test performance for older non-Hispanic White and Black/African American adults. Neuropsychology 2019;33(8):1089.
54. Thames AD, Hinkin CH, Byrd DA, et al. Effects of stereotype threat, perceived discrimination, and examiner race on neuropsychological performance: simple as black and white? J Int Neuropsychological Soc 2013;19(5):583–93.
55. Manly JJ, Echemendia RJ. Race-specific norms: using the model of hypertension to understand issues of race, culture, and education in neuropsychology. Arch Clin Neuropsychol 2007;22(3):319–25.
56. Manly JJ, Jacobs DM, Touradji P, et al. Reading level attenuates differences in neuropsychological test performance between African American and White elders. J Int Neuropsychological Soc 2002;8(3):341–8.
57. Glen T, Hostetter G, Roebuck-Spencer TM, et al. Return on investment and value research in neuropsychology: a call to arms. Arch Clin Neuropsychol 2020;35(5):459–68.
58. McGovern RA, Nelp TB, Kelly KM, et al. Predicting cognitive improvement in normal pressure hydrocephalus patients using preoperative neuropsychological testing and cerebrospinal fluid biomarkers. Neurosurgery 2019;85(4):E662–9.
59. Voon V, Kubu C, Krack P, et al. Deep brain stimulation: neuropsychological and neuropsychiatric issues. Movement Disord official J Movement Disord Soc 2006;21(S14):S305–27.
60. Gelb SR, Shapiro R, Thornton W. Predicting medication adherence and employment status following kidney transplant: the relative utility of traditional and everyday cognitive approaches. Neuropsychology 2010;24(4):514.
61. Cormack F, Shipolini A, Awad WI, et al. A meta-analysis of cognitive outcome following coronary artery bypass graft surgery. Neurosci Biobehav Rev 2012;36(9):2118–29.
62. Welmerink DB, Longstreth W Jr, Lyles MF, et al. Cognition and the risk of hospitalization for serious falls in the elderly: results from the Cardiovascular Health Study. Journals Gerontol Ser A: Biomed Sci Med Sci 2010;65(11):1242–9.
63. Greysen SR, Cenzer IS, Auerbach AD, et al. Functional impairment and hospital readmission in Medicare seniors. JAMA Intern Med 2015;175(4):559–65.
64. Lyon D, Lancaster GA, Taylor S, et al. Predicting the likelihood of emergency admission to hospital of older people: development and validation of the Emergency Admission Risk Likelihood Index (EARLI). Fam Pract 2007;24(2):158–67.
65. Marioni RE, Proust-Lima C, Amieva H, et al. Cognitive lifestyle jointly predicts longitudinal cognitive decline and mortality risk. Eur J Epidemiol 2014;29(3):211–9.
66. Donders J. The incremental value of neuropsychological assessment: a critical review. The Clin Neuropsychologist 2020;34(1):56–87.
67. Leto L, Feola M. Cognitive impairment in heart failure patients. J Geriatr Cardiol JGC. 2014;11(4):316.
68. Svendsboe E, Terum T, Testad I, et al. Caregiver burden in family carers of people with dementia with Lewy bodies and Alzheimer's disease. Int J Geriatr Psychiatry 2016;31(9):1075–83.
69. Hu P, Yang Q, Kong L, et al. Relationship between the anxiety/depression and care burden of the major caregiver of stroke patients. Medicine 2018;97(40).

Brain Networks, Clinical Manifestations, and Neuroimaging of Cognitive Disorders

The Role of Computed Tomography (CT), Magnetic Resonance Imaging (MRI), Positron Emission Tomography (PET), and Other Advanced Neuroimaging Tests

Borna Bonakdarpour, MD*, Clara Takarabe, CMP

KEYWORDS

- MRI • Alzheimer disease • Lewy body disease • SPECT • Cerebrovascular disease
- Computed tomography

KEY POINTS

- In this chapter, three neuroimaging tools (structural, functional, ligand-based) are discussed. These techniques help with localization and diagnosis of the underlying causes of cognitive disorders.
- A network-based approach to cognitive symptoms enhances clinical reasoning and facilitates proper choices for neuroimaging techniques.
- Most common neuropathologic etiologies of cognitive disorders are Alzheimer disease, Lewy body disease, cerebrovascular disease, frontotemporal degeneration, and normal pressure hydrocephalus.
- Cerebrovascular diseases can be diagnosed using a structural brain MRI, while to diagnose Alzheimer disease FDG-PET, and Amyloid PET scans may be necessary.
- Lewy body disease can be diagnosed using characteristic findings on FDG-PET and DaT scans.

Mesulam Center for Cognitive Neurology and Alzheimer's Disease, Ken and Ruth Davee Department of Neurology, Northwestern University Feinberg School of Medicine
* Corresponding author. 300 East Superior Street, Tarry 8, Mesulam Center for Cognitive Neurology and Alzheimer's Disease, Chicago, IL 60611.
E-mail address: bbk@northwestern.edu

Clin Geriatr Med 39 (2023) 45–65
https://doi.org/10.1016/j.cger.2022.07.004
0749-0690/23/© 2022 Elsevier Inc. All rights reserved.

geriatric.theclinics.com

INTRODUCTION

Individuals with neurocognitive disorders present with problems of memory loss, language impairment, visuospatial difficulties, perceptual abnormalities, apraxias, attention/executive dysfunction, and behavioral changes. A neuroanatomical approach to cognitive evaluation can reveal structure-based syndromes, which, together with the proper neuroimaging tool, can assist with localization and, in some cases, diagnosis of the underlying cause of the neurocognitive disorder. Neuroimaging tools can assist with better characterization of the neuroanatomical underpinning of clinical syndromes and diagnosis of the underlying cause.

In this article, we briefly discuss imaging modalities used in clinical settings for neuroanatomical characterization and for diagnosis of the underlying disease. We then discuss how each neuroimaging tool can be used in the context of clinical syndromes. The major underlying causes relevant to our discussion include Alzheimer disease (AD), Lewy body (LB) disease, cerebrovascular disease, frontotemporal degeneration, autoimmune diseases, and systemic or metabolic derangements.

MAJOR NEUROIMAGING DIAGNOSTIC TOOLS

Brain imaging plays a significant role in diagnosis and characterization of neurocognitive disorders. When the clinical syndrome of cognitive impairment is determined anatomic localization and the likely underlying diagnosis can be confirmed using structural imaging (eg, cranial computed tomography, magnetic resonance imaging). If structural imaging is indeterminate, functional imaging can be used to better understand the pathophysiology of the disease. Two major functional modalities that are commonly used are fluorodeoxyglucose positron emission tomography (FDG-PET) and single photon emission tomography (SPECT). The latter is less sensitive than FDG-PET, however, when FDG-PET scan cannot be used (eg, due to lack of insurance coverage), SPECT is a good alternative. With the availability of ligand-based imaging since 2011 (dopamine transporters [DaT][1] and Amyloid PET[2]), we are now able to establish a molecular diagnosis and determine the underlying cause in AD and LB disease.

Structural Neuroimaging

Magnetic resonance imaging

Using a strong magnetic field and radio waves, pictures obtained by MRI reflect different concentrations of hydrogen atoms in the abundant water molecules in brain structures. A resolution of about 1 mm^3 and availability of different sequences to obtain information about anatomic details, make brain MRI the first choice for the evaluation of neurocognitive disorders. T1 sequence is the best MRI modality to investigate structural changes within gray matter, white matter, and spinal fluid spaces (eg, ventricles).[3] T2 sequence, specifically Fluid-Attenuated Inversion Recovery (FLAIR) is helpful in identifying cerebrovascular and inflammatory pathologic condition (eg, white matter damage in multiple sclerosis [MS]).[4] In the Gradient Echo sequence, microbleeds of cerebral amyloid angiopathy (CAA), and heavy metal changes in the basal ganglia can be identified. Diffusion-weighted imaging (DWI) MRI sequence has high sensitivity for the diagnosis of acute strokes.

Computed tomography scan

CT scan images are obtained using X-ray equipment. CT scans of the brain have lower resolution than MRI but the latter are usually used to rule out bleeds and get a general sense of brain structure patients cannot tolerate longer MRI acquisition time or have contraindications to undergo an MRI (eg, have a pacemaker). Calcifications are better distinguished using brain CT scans, and therefore, they are preferred when the diagnosis of brain calcification (eg, in Fahr disease) is in question.[5]

Functional Neuroimaging

Metabolic positron emission tomography
PET is a functional imaging technique based on the measurement of emissions from an injected radiotracer. The most common tracer in clinical practice is FDG[6]. FDG is taken in by nerve cells and concentrations of tracer detected by the scanner correlate with metabolic activity of brain tissue. FDG-PET can be used to look for regions with hypometabolism in neurodegenerative diseases such as AD, LB disease, and frontotemporal degeneration (see later discussion). In normal pressure hydrocephalus, cortical FDG-PET signal is usually normal but there may be decreased metabolism within the caudate nuclei.[7]

Single photon emission tomography
SPECT is based on measurement of regional cerebral blood flow (rCBF) using radiotracers such as Technetium (eg, 99mTc-hexamethylpropylene amine oxime). In neurodegenerative diseases, rCBF, which is a marker of neuronal metabolism, is decreased for structures affected by pathologic condition. The pattern of decreased perfusion usually follows the same pattern seen in the FDG-PET scan.

Ligand-Based Imaging

Amyloid positron emission tomography
A fascinating and important development in the 2000s was the introduction of a tracer that can bind to amyloid plaques in brains of patients with AD. This tracer, which is a neutrally charged benzothiazole derived from thioflavin T, was called the Pittsburgh compound B, and the related PET scan referred to as PiB PET.[8] Using the Pittsburg product, distribution of amyloid plaques can be demonstrated in the brain of patients with Alzheimer neuropathology, and a positive Alzheimer pathologic condition diagnosis can often be confirmed, especially in patients aged younger than 65 year. With advanced age, specificity of the Amyloid PET scan decreases, as cognitively normal older adults may also have positive scans.[9] The tracer, however, has a half-life of about 20 minutes, limiting its feasibility and utility in clinical settings. To improve tracer durability,[10] a different compound, florbetapir, was developed. Florbetapir is a radiotracer containing the radionuclide Fluorine-18. Florbetapir has a longer half-life (110 minutes) and stays longer in the brain, allowing for accumulation. The Food and Drug Administration (FDA) cleared florbetapir PET scanning in 2011,[11,12] and since then, it has been clinically available for the diagnosis of Alzheimer pathologic condition.

Dopamine transporter single photon emission tomography scan
The injected ligand in DaT is Ioflupane (^{123}I), which binds to DaT in the striatum. In LB disease (eg, Lewy body dementia [LBD] and Parkinson disease [PD]), the uptake of Ioflupane in the striatum is decreased due to loss of dopaminergic neurons in the substantia nigra. DaT as a diagnostic modality was cleared by FDA in 2011 and is now covered by insurance companies for the diagnosis of LBD and PD. DaT scan has a sensitivity of 77.7% and specificity of 90.5% for LBD.[13,14] DaT scan may become positive in other neurodegenerative diseases that are associated with extrapyramidal impairment such as progressive supranuclear palsy (PSP)[15–18] and corticobasal degeneration (CBD).[19–21]

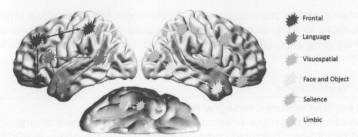

Fig. 1. Basic large-scale brain networks. Red: frontal network has bilateral representations and includes the following major nodes: posterior parietal, frontal eye fields, orbitofrontal cortex. Pink: language network is lateralized to the dominant hemisphere and includes the Broca's, Wernicke's, and anterior temporal nodes. Orange: visuospatial network is lateralized to the right and has the following nodes: posterior parietal and frontal eye fields in the right frontal dorsolateral prefrontal cortex. Yellow: object and face recognition network with main nodes being the fusiform face area and anterior temporal lobe usually on the right side. On the left side, this stream is mostly enmeshed with the naming network. Green: Salience network has bilateral representation with nodes located at anterior insula and orbitofrontal cortex. The social compartmental functions are usually supported by the nondominant hemisphere. Blue: limbic network includes the hippocampus and posterior sphere supporting memory and amygdala and anterior sphere supporting emotions.

What follows is a practical review of major neurocognitive networks and specific imaging findings of different neurocognitive syndromes.

MAJOR NEUROCOGNITIVE NETWORKS

Neurocognitive functions are supported by large-scale brain networks (**Fig. 1**), which are not necessarily confined by cerebral lobar structures. Each network may include nodes that are connected across cerebral lobar organization. For clinical purposes, neurocognitive syndromes can be attributed to at least 6 basic networks that are briefly discussed below. Note that all images are in radiological orientation with the right side of the image representing the patient's left side.

Frontal Executive Network

The frontal network involves 3 regions: the dorsolateral prefrontal, medial prefrontal, and the orbitofrontal cortices. The frontal network is connected to the head of the caudate nucleus and the dorsomedial thalamic nucleus, which are subcortical structures. Combined, these areas govern complex functions of cognition and behavior such as planning, adaptive thinking, and self-control.[22]

Salience Network

The salience network is anchored by the frontoinsular cortices and the paralimbic anterior cingulate cortices, and this network pertains to keeping the individual in homeostasis by selecting external stimuli deserving of our attention.[23]

Visuospatial Network (Dorsal Stream of Visual Processing)

The visuospatial network orients the individual to their external environment via 3 major cortical components: the cingulate cortex, posterior parietal cortex, and the frontal eye field.[22] The visuospatial network allows one to identify visual and spatial relationships among objects.

Language Network

Speech and comprehension of language flows through a distributed network along the perisylvian region of the left language dominant hemisphere. The 3 nodes are Broca's area in the inferior frontal gyrus, Wernicke's area at the parietotemporal junction, and the anterior temporal lobe.[22]

Limbic Network

The limbic network consists of the limbic and the paralimbic areas. The limbic nodes are connected through the hippocampus, amygdala, and the entorhinal cortex, and the paralimbic nodes are connected through the cingulate gyrus, insula, temporopolar cortex, and parts of the orbitofrontal cortex. In addition, the hypothalamus, the anterior and medial nuclei of the thalamus, and the medial and basal section of the striatum constitute a distributed network of the limbic network.[22] The limbic network mediates a complex set of behavioral and emotional responses.

Face and Object Recognition Network (Ventral Stream of Visual Processing)

Object and face processing involves the fusiform gyrus and the anterior and inferior temporal cortex. This network uses the ventral stream of visual processing.[22]

MAJOR NEUROCOGNITIVE SYNDROMES AND THE ROLE OF NEUROIMAGING IN DIAGNOSIS
Inattention and Executive Dysfunction (Frontal Network)

Bilateral frontal lobes are known to support executive function, which possess many components: working memory, control/inhibition, set shift, fluency, reasoning, and vehemence or drive to accomplish tasks.[24] These functions usually localize not only to the frontal lobes but also to the structures that heavily project into the frontal lobes, including bilateral parietal lobes, basal ganglia, reticular activation system, and brain stem.[25,26] Neuropathologic differential diagnosis in these cases involve AD, cerebrovascular disease, frontotemporal lobar degeneration (FTLD), LBD, Normal pressure hydrocephalus (NPH),[27] Fahr disease,[28] and Huntington disease,[29] among others. Patients with pure executive dysfunction may have memory difficulties due to weak encoding and retrieval of information. However, once information is registered, unlike individuals with an amnestic syndrome, they do not lose information as evidenced by intact recognition.

Cerebrovascular disease

Patients with vascular risk factors (hypertension, diabetes mellitus, hypercholesterolemia) and multiple strategic strokes (atherosclerotic or embolic) may develop progressive nonamnestic neurocognitive decline (vascular cognitive impairment) with impairment in attention, executive function, and slowed processing. This can be in the form of cortical, subcortical, lacunar strokes (T2 hypointensity usually surrounded by hyperintense fibrotic tissue), or T2 hyperintensities (**Fig. 2**). In older individuals with vascular cognitive impairment, dual cerebrovascular and AD pathologic conditions are more likely leading to a diagnosis of mixed vascular and Alzheimer neurocognitive disorder. While reviewing scans from this population, attention to signs of neurodegeneration is, therefore, important.

Normal pressure hydrocephalus

Clinical features of NPH include urinary incontinence, gait and balance dysfunction, and a dysexecutive/nonamnestic pattern of neurocognitive disorder. Early diagnosis of NPH is important because it can be reversed with surgical intervention and shunt

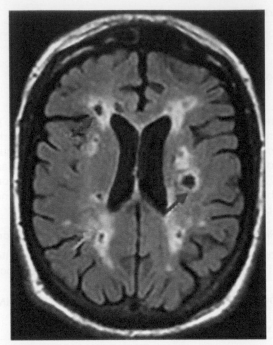

Fig. 2. Cerebrovascular disease: T2 FLAIR MRI: Note subcortical lacunar strokes (*red arrows*), and T2 hyperintensities (*blue arrow*).

placement. Main brain MRI features include dilatation of ventricles, CSF entrapment, widened sylvian fissure, periventricular effusion, and thinning of corpus callosum (**Fig. 3**). FDG-PET scan can help to determine presence or absence of concomitant neurodegenerative disease as cortical metabolism is usually intact in NPH. FDG-PET scan in NPH may show decreased metabolism in the striatum.

Ventriculomegaly characterizes NPH and calculating the Evans' index (EI) and the callosal angle (CA) through MRI is of diagnostic value. The CA can aid in differentiating between NPH and hydrocephalus ex vacuo. The EI is defined as the ratio between the widest diameter of the frontal horns and the maximum inner diameter of the skull in the same axial plane. Usually, a threshold of 0.3 is used. CA is measured in the coronal

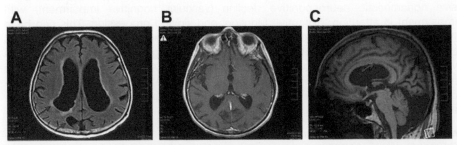

Fig. 3. Normal pressure hydrocephalus: (*A*) Note enlarged ventricles, transependymal effusion, and CSF entrapment (*red arrows*); (*B*) red arrow points to enlargement of the sylvian fissure; and (*C*) corpus callosum thinning (*red arrow*).

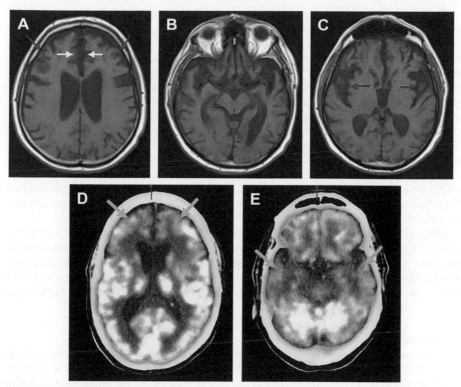

Fig. 4. Frontotemporal degeneration. Note arrows signifying bilateral frontal (red and yellow) (A) temporal (red) (B), and perisylvian (red) (C) atrophy. FDG-PET scan shows bilateral hypometabolism in frontal (D) and temporal lobes (E) as shown by blue arrows.

plane through the posterior commissure perpendicular to the AC-PC plane. It usually ranges between 50° and 80° in NPH, and this angle is smaller compared with hydrocephalus ex vacuo.[30]

Frontotemporal lobar degeneration

FTLD is an umbrella term for a large number of conditions that commonly have the tendency to affect the frontal and temporal lobes. However, these conditions can also affect the parietal and limbic regions as well. They can be bilateral or asymmetric, and they may or may not be associated with motor disorders such as motor neuron disease or Parkinsonism (CBD and PSP). All these conditions are caused by the accumulation of abnormal inclusions in brain cells that are made of abnormal tau protein or Tar DNA-binding protein 43. The phenotypic presentation of FTLDs includes behavioral variant frontotemporal dementia (bvFTD), corticobasal syndrome (CBS), PSP syndrome, nonfluent/agrammatic primary progressive aphasia (nfaPPA), and semantic variant PPA. The last 2 categories will be discussed under language disorders.

Patients with bvFTD, in addition to executive dysfunction, can present with impulsivity, poor judgment, and lack of insight, apathy, and inappropriate social behaviors. Brain MRI shows atrophy in the frontal lobes that may involve dorsolateral prefrontal cortex (executive dysfunction), mesial frontal cortex (apathy, abulia), and orbitofrontal cortex (impulsivity; **Fig. 4**).

Progressive supranuclear palsy is caused by frontotemporal degeneration with 4-repeat tau inclusions accumulating as tufted astrocytes.[31] Phenotypes presenting primarily with cognitive disorder are mostly seen in cognitive neurology clinics in contrast to phenotypes with extrapyramidal derangements. These phenotypes include frontal type neurocognitive disorder, nfaPPA, primary progressive apraxia of speech/dysarthria, and motoric phenotype known as Richardson syndrome (vertical gaze palsy, gait instability and falls, and Parkinsonian rigidity). Neuroanatomical features that can differentiate these groups of conditions from other frontal type neurocognitive disorders are related to changes in the midbrain. Cerebral peduncles become prominent due to atrophy within the midbrain tegmentum, which can be seen on axial MRI or CT scans, known also as the Mickey Mouse sign (**Fig. 5**A). Concave atrophy of the midbrain on sagittal view, and its narrowing toward the optic chiasm gives the midbrain a look known as "Hummingbird sign" (**Fig. 5**B). A ratio of midbrain to pons less than 0.52 has 100% specificity to differentiate PSP from multiple system atrophy and PD.[32]

CBD, similar to PSP, is caused by 4-repeat tau inclusions formed as astrocytic plaques.[31] CBD can present with an FTD syndrome with Parkinsonism; however, it tends to affect brain hemispheres asymmetrically (CBS). In right-handed individuals, right hemisphere dominant pathologic condition will cause visuospatial disturbances and left-sided limb apraxia, whereas left-sided lesions cause aphasia and right-sided limb rigidity and apraxia (**Fig. 6**).

Fahr disease
Fahr disease is a rare familial autosomal dominant or recessive or idiopathic calcification of the basal ganglia (**Fig. 7**). The clinical presentation of Fahr disease is the progressive decline of psychiatric, cognitive, and/or neurologic (ie, seizures, cerebellar impairment, speech impairment, or extrapyramidal disorder) function. The psychiatric presentation first manifests on a spectrum ranging from mild difficulty with concentration and memory, to changes in personality or behavior, to psychosis and dementia in

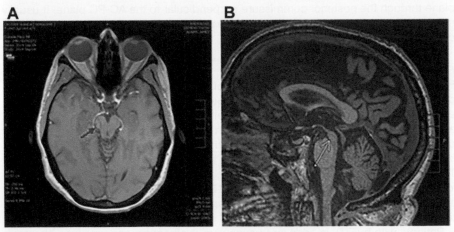

Fig. 5. Progressive supranuclear palsy. (*A*) Brain axial view: Red arrow shows prominence of cerebral peduncles due to atrophy of midbrain tegmentum (Mickey Mouse sign). (*B*) Brain sagittal view: Red arrow shows thinning of midbrain (Hummingbird sign). White arrow indicates the diagonal diameter of pons. Note that midbrain tegmentum is less than half the pontine base.

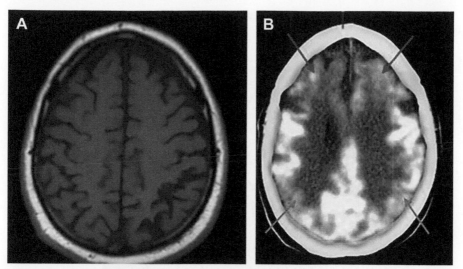

Fig. 6. Corticobasal degeneration. (*A*) Axial brain MRI: 49-year-old man with CBS and right-hand apraxia. (*B*) Axial FDG-PET scan: 58-year-old man with FTD (apathy, executive dysfunction), falls, and right-sided extrapyramidal symptoms (CBS). Red arrows indicate hypometabolism in the frontal lobes. Blue arrows indicate hypometabolism in the bilateral parietal lobes.

severe cases. Extrapyramidal symptoms can include tremors, gait disturbances, parkinsonism, and dystonia. Fahr disease is associated with extensive calcification often involving the cerebral sulci, basal ganglia, dentate nucleus, subthalamic nucleus, red nucleus, and other regions. Deposits accumulate in the walls of capillaries, arterioles, and small veins, and in perivascular spaces and pericytes. Intimal fibrosis and narrowing may occur. Surrounding these regions of calcification is neuronal degeneration, gliosis and reduced cerebral blood flow. The imaging-based criterion is bilateral

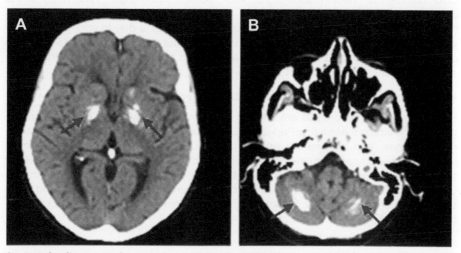

Fig. 7. Fahr disease. Red arrows point to basal ganglia (*A*) and cerebellar dentate nuclei (*B*) calcifications.

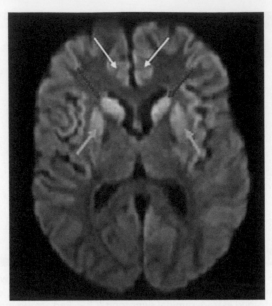

Fig. 8. Creutzfeldt Jakob disease. Axial MRI DWI sequence shows hyperintensities within the basal ganglia (blue: putamen, and red: head of caudate), also known as hockey stick sign. Yellow arrows point to "cortical ribboning" within mesial frontal regions.

striopallidodentate calcification, which is best detected with CT scan. A cloudy thin linear appearance has high specificity for Fahr disease, and massive calcification has moderate specificity. On T2-weighted MRI, there is often a hyperintense signal in the basal ganglia.

Creutzfeldt Jakob disease

CJD is caused by prion disease and usually presents with a confusional state associated with myoclonus and extrapyramidal symptoms.[33] Characteristic MRI findings of CJD include the "hockey stick sign," and "cortical ribboning."[34] The head of the caudate nucleus constitutes the head of the hockey stick and the handle is due to hyperintensity of the putamen (**Fig. 8**). Cortical ribboning is due to spongiform injury within the cortex. It is important to note that the clinical syndrome depends on where cortical injury is localized. As noted later, an aphasic or visual agnostic syndrome can also be primary presentations of CJD.

Memory Loss and Amnestic Syndromes (Limbic Network)

Primary amnestic syndromes are caused by neuropathology within the posterior regions of the limbic system (the Papez circuit) including the hippocampus, fornix, anterior thalamus, and mammillary bodies. Individuals with neuropathology in these regions will have short-term memory loss with difficulty in retention and lack of ability to recognize items they learned. Differential diagnosis of an amnestic syndrome includes AD, Wernicke-Korsakoff encephalopathy, cerebrovascular disease, and other pathologic conditions that can affect the limbic system (eg, MS) may cause an amnestic syndrome.

Alzheimer disease

In the presence of Alzheimer pathologic condition, 90% of patients present with typical amnestic syndrome.[35] Typically, individuals with amnestic Alzheimer syndrome

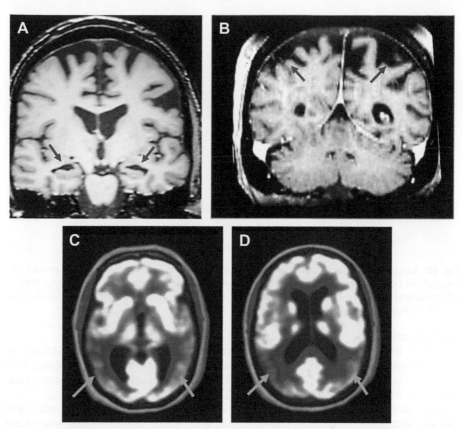

Fig. 9. Typical Alzheimer disease. Top row: Coronal slices: note red arrows pointing to hippocampal (*A*) and parietal (*B*) atrophy. Bottom row: Axial FDG-PET slices show bilateral temporal (*C*) and parietotemporal (*D*) hypometabolism (*blue arrows*).

have difficulty with retention of information while encoding of information is not usually impaired until later stages of the disease. Major regions of atrophy in typical AD include the bilateral hippocampi, and the association cortices of the parietal lobes and perisylvian regions. Frontal lobes are involved later and primary sensory and motor cortices are usually not affected by AD (**Fig. 9**A, B). During earlier stages of typical AD, atrophy may not be significant. In these cases, FDG-PET may reveal hypometabolism in the bilateral parietotemporal regions (**Fig. 9**C, D).[36,37]

Based on clinical syndromology, an amnestic syndrome is due to an underlying Alzheimer pathologic condition only in 88% of cases, vascular injuries being another common cause. Therefore, for more accurate diagnosis of the underlying cause, additional workup may be needed. Evaluation of the spinal fluid for beta amyloid and tau proteins is now becoming a standard part of the workup for neurocognitive disorder; however, because it is an invasive procedure, it may not be a favorable approach, especially in cases when the patient is on anticoagulants. Amyloid PET scan provides an alternative in such cases, although unfortunately it is not yet covered by insurance companies. In patients with AD, the border zone between the white and gray matter is less visible on the amyloid PET and both tend to bind with tagged amyloid tracers (**Fig. 10**). As mentioned earlier, it is important to bear in mind that 10% to 20% of asymptomatic adults aged older than 65 years may have positive amyloid scans.

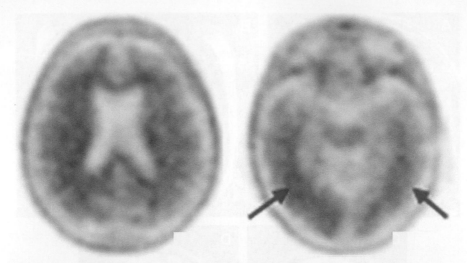

Fig. 10. Amyloid PET scan in a patient with Alzheimer disease. The tracer is seen in dark color and the border zone between the white and gray matter is not well seen, except for the left temporal lobe (*red arrow*), which provides a good comparison between normal looking and abnormal regions.

Multiple sclerosis

Structural lesions within different components of the Papez circuit can cause an amnestic syndrome resembling what is usually seen in Alzheimer type neurocognitive disorder. For example, MS plaques can affect the fornix causing limbic memory loss, which can occasionally be seen in MS (**Fig. 11**) [REF].[38,39]

Heavy alcohol use in the form of binge drinking can cause thiamine deficiency and damage within the mammillary bodies, fornix, and medial thalamic nuclei and cause symptoms of confusion, amnestic cognitive impairment, gaze palsy, and ataxia (**Fig. 12**).[40]

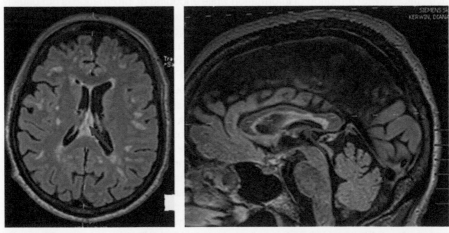

Fig. 11. Multiple sclerosis. T2 FLAIR images. Note hyperintensity within the fornix on both axial (left red arrow) and sagittal (right red arrow) views representing plaques affecting the fornix causing an amnestic syndrome.

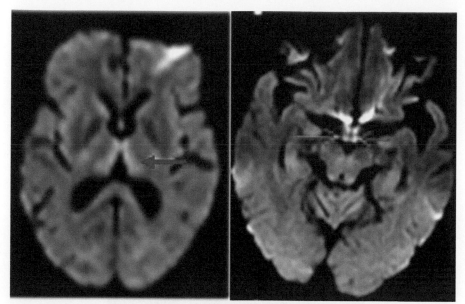

Fig. 12. Wernicke encephalopathy. T2 FLAIR. Red arrow shows hyperintensity within the mediodorsal thalamic nuclei. Green arrows point to mammillary body hyperintensities signifying necrosis in that region.

Aphasic Syndromes (Dominant Perisylvian Language Network)

In 99% of right-handed individuals, language is processed in the left hemisphere. In left-handed persons, language is lateralized to the left hemisphere in 70% of cases, right hemisphere in 15% of cases, and has bilateral representations in another 15% of cases.[41] Any brain pathologic condition that affects the perisylvian language zone of the brain can cause aphasia (eg, stroke, neoplasms, neurodegenerative diseases, traumatic brain injury, focal inflammatory injuries due to sarcoidosis or vasculitis, herpes encephalitis).

Cerebrovascular disease and stroke

The most common cause of aphasia is cerebrovascular disease and stroke. In individuals with advanced age and chronic stroke worsening of symptoms is possible due to trans-synaptic degeneration and age or Alzheimer-related neurodegeneration **(Fig. 13)**.[42]

CAA is caused by amyloid deposition within cerebral vasculature, which makes them prone to blood leakage, microhemorrhages, and, in severe cases, acute lobar hemorrhage. Chronic microbleeds, inflammation, and ischemia can cause damage to the subcortical white matter, especially in posterior occipito-temporal regions.[43,44] In cases with asymmetric dominant hemisphere lesions, patients can present with an anomic/aphasic syndrome **(Fig. 14)**.

Neurodegenerative diseases

Language network can be affected by neurodegenerative diseases in a primary or nonprimary fashion. In primary progressive aphasias (PPA), aphasia is the only cognitive impairment for at least a year before other cognitive domains are affected. Aphasia, however, remains the major disability in these patients. In nonprimary form,

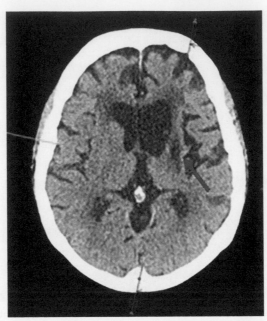

Fig. 13. Chronic stroke and superimposing neurodegenerative changes. The patient had a CT scan because she had a pacemaker, making her ineligible for an MRI. Note left subinsular stroke (*thick red arrow*), white matter vascular injuries (*blue arrows*) and neurodegenerative changes and atrophy (*thin red arrow*), which is more severe on the side of the stroke.

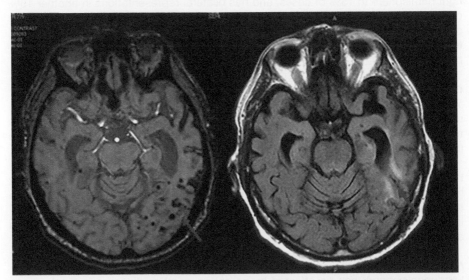

Fig. 14. Cerebral amyloid angiopathy. Red arrows show areas of microvascular bleeds in the GRE axial MRI sequence (A) and white matter hyperintensities in this T2 FLAIR sequence. In this patient, lesions are asymmetrically affecting the left temporo-occipital lobe causing visual and anomic disturbances.

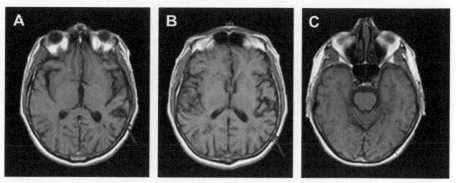

Fig. 15. Logopenic primary progressive aphasia (PPA-L). Red arrow shows areas of atrophy in the left parietotemporal region (*A, B*). Note that there is no atrophy in the bilateral hippocampi, in contrast to typical AD (*C*).

aphasia is only a part of a multidomain neurocognitive disorder. Two major causes of PPA include AD and frontotemporal degeneration. There have also been reports of leukodystrophies,[45] CJD[46,47] causing PPA. LB disease is commonly (up to 40% of cases) associated with concomitant Alzheimer pathologic condition. In some cases, AD may cause progressive aphasia complicating the picture of LB disease.[48] Very occasionally, LB disease can also cause an anomic/logopenic pattern of aphasia.[49]

Alzheimer disease: As mentioned above, 10% of AD patients present as nonamnestic syndromes. The most common form of aphasic AD is logopenic variant PPA (PPA-L or lvPPA). Individuals with PPA-L have word finding pauses, circumlocutions, anomia, and difficulty with repetition of sentences. The pathologic hallmark of PPA-L is plaques and tangles in the temporoparietal junction, which can be seen as atrophy in structural imaging and hypometabolism or hypoperfusion in function neuroimaging (**Fig. 15**). In rarer cases, AD can cause overly nonfluent/agrammatic PPA (PPA-G or nfaPPA).

FTLD: Both forms of FTLD pathologic condition (tau and TDP43) can present with PPA-G where there is mostly atrophy in the dominant inferior frontal lobe, extending to dorsal premotor areas (**Fig. 16**). Semantic variant of PPA (PPA-S), is specifically associated with FTLD-TDP43-C neuropathology and specifically affects the anterior

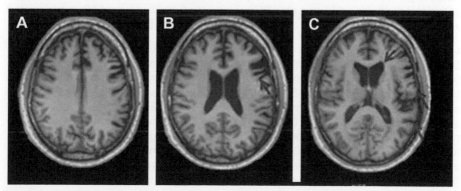

Fig. 16. Nonfluent/agrammatic primary progressive aphasia (PPA-G). Note atrophy within the left frontal (*A, B*), and perisylvian regions (*C*). There is increased size of the left lateral ventricular horn (*C*).

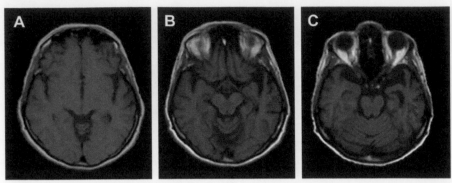

Fig. 17. Semantic primary progressive aphasia (PPA-S). Axial MR images: Note normal appearance of the perisylvian regions (*A*). Red arrows show atrophy within the left anterior temporal lobe (*B, C*).

temporal lobes (ATLs) in early stages (left > right; **Fig. 17**). In the beginning, the patient has significant difficulty with naming objects, and then they have additional weakness in understanding single words. When both ATLs have undergone neurodegeneration, the patient will have difficulty with recognizing objects and faces. At that point, this condition is called semantic dementia.

Visuospatial Impairment (Nondominant Parietofrontal Network)

Advanced visual processing in the brain can be affected by many underlying causes including stroke, neurodegenerative disease (AD, LB disease, CBD), infections (CJD), neoplasms, and traumatic brain injury, among others. Patients may have trouble with spatial navigation, simultanagnosia, optic ataxia, oculomotor apraxia (Balint syndrome), dressing apraxia, or agraphia, acalculia, finger agnosia, and left–right disorientation (Gerstmann syndrome). If both of the latter syndromes are present a clinical diagnosis of posterior cortical atrophy (PCA) is used to describe the clinical picture.[50]

Alzheimer disease

Visual processing abnormalities and agnosias can be part of the amnestic Alzheimer's neurocognitive disorder or may start as primary presentation of the disease, usually in younger individuals (<65 years old). PCA syndrome (visual variant of AD) is associated with significant atrophy within the bilateral parietal lobes (**Fig. 18**).

Lewy body disease

LB disease is another cause of visual processing disturbances. Symptoms resemble those caused by AD. In addition, patients also have extrapyramidal symptoms such as bradykinesia, axial rigidity and falls, and REM behavior disorder. In LB disease, frontal executive functions are also impaired due to the close relationship between parietal and frontal lobes (see **Fig. 1**). Compared with AD, LB disease is not associated with much cortical atrophy. Therefore, functional neuroimaging techniques are more helpful in diagnosis of LB disease. On DaT scan, there is evidence for decreased DaT binding (**Fig. 19**B). On FDG-PET evaluation, LBD patients have decreased metabolism in the biparietal cortices. However, contrary to AD, there is no decrease in posterior cingulate cortex metabolism. As metabolism in the occipital cortex is also decreased in LBD, cingulate cortex is seen as a bright island, hence "cingulate island sign" (**Fig. 19**).

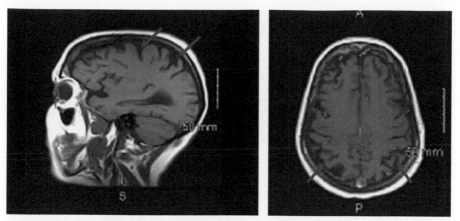

Fig. 18. Posterior cortical atrophy. Red arrows in the sagittal (*left*) and axial (*right*) T1 images point to areas of parietal atrophy.

Creutzfeldt Jakob disease

Creutzfeldt Jakob disease (CJD) can affect association cortices of the parietal lobes and cause a PCA syndrome. This variant of CJD is called the Heidenhain variant.[51] In this case, the disease progresses in a rapid case, which distinguishes it from AD and LBD. On MRI DWI sequence, cortical ribboning can be seen in the bilateral parietal cortices.

Face and Object Agnosias (Ventral Visual Stream)

Lesions affecting the ventral stream of visual processing within the nondominant hemisphere can cause object agnosia and prosopagnosia (impaired face recognition). This can happen in the context of a posterior cerebral artery stroke (**Fig. 20**) in patients with FTLD-TDP43-C type.[52]

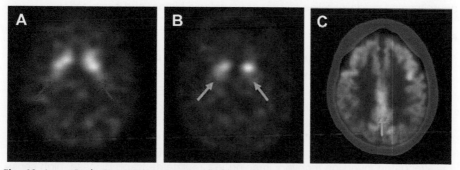

Fig. 19. Lewy Body Dementia. DaT scan (left): In (*A*), DaT scan reveals inverse comma-like structures normal basal ganglia tracer uptake, which is normal (*red arrows*). In (*B*), there is decrease in bilateral basal ganglia tracer uptake (*blue arrows*) signifying the presence of Lewy body disease. FDG-PET scan (*C*) shows decreased metabolism in the parietal and occipital lobes but preserving posterior cingulate region (Cingulate Island sign).

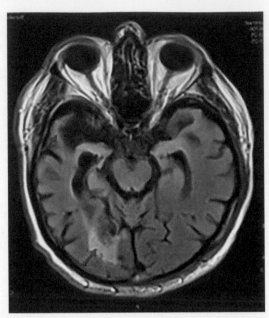

Fig. 20. Posterior cerebral artery territory stroke and neurodegeneration. Note encephalomalacia within the right occipital and temporal lobe and also concomitant atrophy in the temporal lobe (*red arrows*).

SUMMARY

In this article, we reviewed how major neuroimaging tools including CT scan, MRI (structural neuroimaging), FDG-PET, SPECT (functional neuroimaging), and amyloid PET, DaT scan (ligand-based neuroimaging) can help with localization and diagnosis of the underlying cause in neurocognitive disorders. Major neurocognitive networks, their abnormalities, and differential diagnosis of their pathologic condition were discussed. We also demonstrated characteristic neuroimaging findings for each pathologic condition within a certain neurocognitive network. It is important to remember that neuroimaging is an extension of clinical evaluation and that choice of appropriate neuroimaging modality relies on proper neurologic history and examination.

REFERENCES

1. Cooper CA, Chahine LM. Biomarkers in Prodromal Parkinson disease: a Qualitative review. J Int Neuropsychol Soc 2016;22(10):956–67.
2. Cohen AD, Landau SM, Snitz BE, et al. Fluid and PET biomarkers for amyloid pathology in Alzheimer's disease. Mol Cell Neurosci 2019;97:3–17.
3. Desikan RS, Rafii MS, Brewer JB, et al. An expanded role for neuroimaging in the evaluation of memory impairment. AJNR Am J Neuroradiol 2013;34(11):2075–82.
4. Young GS, Geschwind MD, Fischbein NJ, et al. Diffusion-weighted and fluid-attenuated inversion recovery imaging in Creutzfeldt-Jakob disease: high sensitivity and specificity for diagnosis. AJNR Am J Neuroradiol 2005;26(6):1551–62.
5. Runge VM, Aoki S, Bradley WG Jr, et al. Magnetic resonance imaging and computed tomography of the brain—50 Years of Innovation, with a Focus on the Future. Invest Radiol 2015;50(9):551.

6. Singhal T, Narayanan TK, Jacobs MP, et al. 11C-methionine PET for grading and prognostication in gliomas: a comparison study with 18F-FDG PET and contrast enhancement on MRI. J Nucl Med 2012;53(11):1709–15.
7. Graff-Radford NR, Jones DT. Normal Press Hydrocephalus. *Continuum* . 2019; 25(1):165–86.
8. Klunk WE, Engler H, Nordberg A, et al. Imaging brain amyloid in Alzheimer's disease with Pittsburgh Compound-B. Ann Neurol 2004;55(3):306–19.
9. Johnson KA, Minoshima S, Bohnen NI, et al. Appropriate use criteria for amyloid PET: a report of the amyloid imaging task Force, the Society of nuclear Medicine and molecular imaging, and the Alzheimer's association. Alzheimers Dement 2013;9(1):e.1-16.
10. Wong DF, Rosenberg PB, Zhou Y, et al. In vivo imaging of amyloid deposition in Alzheimer disease using the radioligand 18F-AV-45 (florbetapir [corrected] F 18). J Nucl Med 2010;51(6):913–20.
11. Carome M, Wolfe S. Florbetapir-PET imaging and postmortem beta-amyloid pathology. JAMA 2011;305(18):1857 [author reply: 1857–8].
12. Clark CM, Schneider JA, Bedell BJ, et al. Use of florbetapir-PET for imaging beta-amyloid pathology. JAMA 2011;305(3):275–83.
13. McKeith I, O'Brien J, Walker Z, et al. Sensitivity and specificity of dopamine transporter imaging with 123I-FP-CIT SPECT in dementia with Lewy bodies: a phase III, multicentre study. Lancet Neurol 2007;6(4):305–13.
14. Nihashi T, Ito K, Terasawa T. Diagnostic accuracy of DAT-SPECT and MIBG scintigraphy for dementia with Lewy bodies: an updated systematic review and Bayesian latent class model meta-analysis. Eur J Nucl Med Mol Imaging 2020; 47(8):1984–97.
15. Ilgin N, Zubieta J, Reich SG, et al. PET imaging of the dopamine transporter in progressive supranuclear palsy and Parkinson's disease. Neurology 1999; 52(6):1221–6.
16. Sakamoto F, Shiraishi S, Kitajima M, et al. Diagnostic performance of 123I-FPCIT SPECT specific binding ratio in progressive supranuclear palsy: use of core clinical features and MRI for comparison. AJR Am J Roentgenol 2020;215(6):1443–8.
17. Takaya S, Sawamoto N, Okada T, et al. Differential diagnosis of parkinsonian syndromes using dopamine transporter and perfusion SPECT. Parkinsonism Relat Disord 2018;47:15–21.
18. Seppi K, Scherfler C, Donnemiller E, et al. Topography of dopamine transporter availability in progressive supranuclear palsy: a voxelwise [123I]beta-CIT SPECT analysis. Arch Neurol 2006;63(8):1154–60.
19. Booth TC, Nathan M, Waldman AD, et al. The role of functional dopamine-transporter SPECT imaging in parkinsonian syndromes, part 1. AJNR Am J Neuroradiol 2015;36(2):229–35.
20. Cilia R, Rossi C, Frosini D, et al. Dopamine transporter SPECT imaging in corticobasal syndrome. PLoS One 2011;6(5):e18301.
21. Ogawa T, Fujii S, Kuya K, et al. Role of neuroimaging on differentiation of Parkinson's disease and its related diseases. Yonago Acta Med 2018;61(3):145–55.
22. Mesulam. Aphasia, memory loss, and other focal cerebral disorders. Harrison's Principles of Internal Medicine. 21st edition 2022. in press.
23. Seeley WW, Menon V, Schatzberg AF, et al. Dissociable intrinsic connectivity networks for salience processing and executive control. J Neurosci 2007;27(9): 2349–56.
24. Rabinovici GD, Stephens ML, Possin KL. Executive dysfunction. Continuum 2015;21(3 Behavioral Neurology and Neuropsychiatry):646–59.

25. Mesulam M. Representation, inference, and transcendent encoding in neurocognitive networks of the human brain. Ann Neurol 2008;64(4):367–78.
26. Loscalzo J, Fauci AS, Kasper DL, et al. Harrison's principles of internal Medicine. New York: McGraw Hill; 2022.
27. Capone PM, Bertelson JA, Ajtai B. Neuroimaging of normal pressure hydrocephalus and hydrocephalus. Neurol Clin 2020;38(1):171–83.
28. Faria AV, Pereira IC, Nanni L. Computerized tomography findings in Fahr's syndrome. Arq Neuropsiquiatr 2004;62(3B):789–92.
29. Johnson EB, Gregory S. Huntington's disease: brain imaging in Huntington's disease. Prog Mol Biol Transl Sci 2019;165:321–69.
30. Staffaroni AM, Elahi FM, McDermott D, et al. Neuroimaging in dementia. Semin Neurol 2017;37(5):510–37.
31. VandeVrede L, Ljubenkov PA, Rojas JC, et al. Four-repeat tauopathies: current Management and Future treatments. Neurotherapeutics 2020;17(4):1563–81.
32. Massey LA, Jäger HR, Paviour DC, et al. The midbrain to pons ratio: a simple and specific MRI sign of progressive supranuclear palsy. Neurology 2013;80(20): 1856–61.
33. Geschwind MD. Rapidly progressive dementia. Continuum 2016;22(2 Dementia): 510–37.
34. Collie DA, Sellar RJ, Zeidler M, et al. MRI of Creutzfeldt-Jakob disease: imaging features and recommended MRI protocol. Clin Radiol 2001;56(9):726–39.
35. Murray ME, Graff-Radford NR, Ross OA, et al. Neuropathologically defined subtypes of Alzheimer's disease with distinct clinical characteristics: a retrospective study. Lancet Neurol 2011;10(9):785–96.
36. Langbaum JBS, Chen K, Lee W, et al. Categorical and correlational analyses of baseline fluorodeoxyglucose positron emission tomography images from the Alzheimer's Disease Neuroimaging Initiative (ADNI). Neuroimage 2009;45(4): 1107–16.
37. Kawachi T, Ishii K, Sakamoto S, et al. Comparison of the diagnostic performance of FDG-PET and VBM-MRI in very mild Alzheimer's disease. Eur J Nucl Med Mol Imaging 2006;33(7):801–9.
38. Basso MR, Whiteside D, Combs D, et al. Memory in multiple sclerosis: a reappraisal using the item specific deficit approach. Neuropsychology 2021;35(2): 207–19.
39. Syc SB, Harrison DM, Saidha S, et al. Quantitative MRI demonstrates abnormality of the fornix and cingulum in multiple sclerosis. Mult Scler Int 2013;2013:838719.
40. Sullivan EV, Pfefferbaum A. Neuroimaging of the Wernicke-Korsakoff syndrome. Alcohol Alcohol 2009;44(2):155–65.
41. Helm-Estabrooks N, Albert ML, Nicholas M. Manual of aphasia and aphasia Therapy. New York: PRO-ED; 2014.
42. Ellis C, Urban S. Age and aphasia: a review of presence, type, recovery and clinical outcomes. Top Stroke Rehabil 2016;23(6):430–9.
43. Wardlaw JM, Smith C, Dichgans M. Small vessel disease: mechanisms and clinical implications. Lancet Neurol 2019;18(7):684–96.
44. Jiang L, Cai X, Yao D, et al. Association of inflammatory markers with cerebral small vessel disease in community-based population. J Neuroinflammation 2022;19(1):106.
45. Oboudiyat C, Bigio EH, Bonakdarpour B, et al. Diffuse leukoencephalopathy with spheroids presenting as primary progressive aphasia. Neurology 2015;85(7): 652–3.

46. Balash Y, Korczyn AD, Khmelev N, et al. Creutzfeldt-jakob and vascular brain diseases: their Overlap and relationships. Front Neurol 2021;12:613991.
47. Mahboob HB, Kaokaf KH, Gonda JM. Creutzfeldt-jakob disease presenting as expressive aphasia and nonconvulsive Status epilepticus. Case Rep Crit Care 2018;2018:5053175.
48. Apple AC, Mao Q, Bigio E, et al. Sleep talking and primary progressive aphasia: case study and autopsy findings in a patient with logopenic primary progressive aphasia and dementia with Lewy bodies. BMJ Case Rep 2019;12(5). https://doi.org/10.1136/bcr-2018-228938.
49. Watanabe H, Ikeda M, Mori E. Primary progressive aphasia as a Prodromal state of dementia with Lewy bodies: a case report. Front Neurol 2020;11. https://doi.org/10.3389/fneur.2020.00049.
50. Mendez MF. Early-onset Alzheimer disease and its variants. Continuum 2019;25(1):34–51.
51. Manners DN, Parchi P, Tonon C, et al. Pathologic correlates of diffusion MRI changes in Creutzfeldt-Jakob disease. Neurology 2009;72(16):1425–31.
52. Pelak VS. The clinical approach to the identification of higher-order visual dysfunction in neurodegenerative disease. Curr Neurol Neurosci Rep 2022;22(4):229–42.

Blood and Cerebrospinal Fluid Biomarkers in Vascular Dementia and Alzheimer's Disease
A Brief Review

Philip B. Gorelick, MD, MPH

KEYWORDS

• Biomarkers • Blood • Cerebrospinal fluid (CSF) • Amyloid beta (Aβ) • Tau

KEY POINTS

- A biomarker is as an indicator of normal biological processes, pathogenic processes, or responses to an exposure or intervention.
- Biomarkers for the dementias are primarily a research tool that has more recently begun to be utilized in clinical practice.
- Key biomarkers for Alzheimer's disease include cerebrospinal fluid and blood measures of amyloid beta (Aβ) and tau, and Aβ-PET, tau-PET, and fluorodeoxyglucose-PET scan measures.
- Elucidation of key fluid and other biomarkers for vascular cognitive impairment are currently under study.
- Biomarkers must be interpreted within the context of the clinical dementia phenotype.

INTRODUCTION

The maintenance of brain health is a lifelong process whereby potentially deleterious exposures such as cardiovascular risks, amyloid beta (Aβ), and phosphorylated tau (p-tau) may adversely affect the brain decades before there are clinical manifestations.[1,2] Thus, the early structural and neuropathological foundation for the development of cognitive impairment and its allied features later in life may provide precursor targets such that interventions may be applied to prevent or slow cognitively impairing processes if the underlying mechanism(s) can be addressed in time. In addition, there seems to be a reciprocal relationship between cerebrovascular disease, a currently preventable and modifiable disorder, and neurodegeneration. In fact, one of the earliest changes in

Section of Stroke and Neurocritical Care, Davee Department of Neurology, Northwestern University Feinberg School of Medicine, 625 North Michigan Avenue Suite 1150, Chicago, IL 60611, USA
E-mail address: philip.gorelick@gmail.com

Clin Geriatr Med 39 (2023) 67–76
https://doi.org/10.1016/j.cger.2022.08.001
0749-0690/23/© 2022 Elsevier Inc. All rights reserved.

geriatric.theclinics.com

Alzheimer's disease (AD) may be dysfunction of the blood–brain barrier leading to alterations in cerebral blood flow.[2] Vascular dysfunction in AD has been referred to as a potentially important but "disregarded partner."[3] As such vascular advocates have argued that vascular biomarkers should be incorporated into the AD research framework.[3] In 2018, the US National Institutes of Health (NIH) introduced a new research framework moving the definition of AD from clinical consequences of disease (ie, signs and symptoms) to a biological construct.[4] Specifically, the new focus for the diagnosis of AD included biomarkers grouped according to the following scheme: ATN (A for Aβ accumulation in the brain; T for tau deposits; and N for neurodegeneration).[4] The proposed research framework has now spilled over into clinical practice where blood and cerebrospinal fluid (CSF) biomarkers are being used by health care providers for the purpose of prevention, diagnosis, and treatment.

In this discussion, the author reviews (1) the definition of a biomarker; (2) common biomarkers to consider in the more frequent causes of dementia, vascular cognitive impairment (VCI) or vascular cognitive disorder (VCD), and AD; and (3) limitations of biomarkers and their clinical relevance in practice. Biomarkers hold promise to improve the diagnosis and care of persons at risk of or who have cognitive impairment, especially in the early stages. In this brief review, the author provides guidance for health care providers who may be considering use of biomarkers in the diagnosis and management of patients with cognitive impairment.

DEFINITION OF A BIOMARKER

In 2016, a US Federal Drug Agency-NIH work group created a source reference text on biomarkers called, BEST (Biomarkers, Endpoints, and Other Tools) Resource.[5] In the reference resource, the following definition of a biomarker was provided: a characteristic that is measured as an indicator of normal biological processes, pathogenic processes, or responses to an exposure or intervention, including therapeutic interventions.[5] In addition, biomarkers were classified by type (molecular, histologic, radiographic, and physiologic) and category (safety, diagnostic, prognostic, monitoring, and others).[5] The reference resource includes other topics of interest such as validation of biomarkers, surrogate endpoints, and biomarker qualification and context of use.[5]

In the domain of dementia and related disorders, underlying mechanisms of cognitive impairment are thought to be linked to factors such as cardiovascular risks, misfolded proteins (eg, Aβ), oxidative stress, and neuroinflammation. Therefore, the focus of biomarker discovery, for example, in AD, has been Aβ, tau, and neuroimaging markers of neuronal degeneration (eg, localized brain atrophy). Underlying biological mechanisms for brain injury in cognitive impairment are reviewed in more detail in Betul Kara and colleagues' article, "Vascular and Non-vascular Mechanisms of Cognitive Impairment and Dementia," in this issue.

BIOMARKERS TO CONSIDER IN COMMON CAUSES OF DEMENTIA
Vascular Cognitive Impairment or Vascular Cognitive Disorder

In the ensuing discussion, the author uses the terms VCI and VCD synonymously as a means to refer to cognitive disorders with mechanistic underpinnings of cerebrovascular disease, although there are nuances which separate the definition of the clinical terms VCI and VCD that are addressed elsewhere.[6] For sake of simplicity of language, the author uses the term VCI going forward.

In the 1970s, Dr Gary Rosenberg, a pioneer in biomarkers for VCI, studied patients with a cerebrovascular condition referred to as subcortical arteriosclerotic encephalopathy of Binswanger.[7] The condition was characterized clinically by subcortical strokes, hypertension, dementia, spasticity, syncope, and seizures, and neuropathologically by diffuse demyelination of brain white matter or foci of necrosis plus arteriosclerotic and hypertensive vasculopathy.[7] In this condition, cranial computed tomography (CT) or MRI of the brain traditionally shows substantial white matter disease (ie, white matter hyperintensities or leukoaraiosis [rarefaction of the white matter]). In the encephalopathy of Binswanger, Rosenberg was one of the clinical scientists to call to attention the possible role of neuroinflammation as a factor underlying damage to cerebral white matter.[8] In addition, he emphasized the potential role of matrix metalloproteinases (MMPs) which may injure (1) tight junctions of the blood–brain barrier leading to leakage of toxic blood compartment components into brain white matter and (2) myelin, leading to a loss of its integrity.[8] These observations helped to establish a foundation for the future application of biomarkers for inflammation and MMPs as mechanistic targets for intervention in persons with cerebral subcortical small vessel disease (SSVD).[8]

There are a number of studies, many of which are small or remain unvalidated, and reviews on the topic of biomarkers for VCI. Some of the research addresses the overlap between VCI and AD. In the realm of VCI, there is considerable interest in SSVD as this condition seems to be the most common form of cerebrovascular disease associated with cognitive impairment. In one review, Wallin and colleagues[9] carried out a comprehensive literature search of biomarkers for VCI-SSVD. Based on their review, common mechanistic themes emerged. There were biomarkers related to disruption of blood-CSF and the blood–brain barrier, breakdown of brain white matter and the extracellular matrix, and blood and brain inflammatory markers.[9] Specifically, elevated CSF/blood albumin ratio, a marker of blood-CSF and blood–brain barrier disruption; altered CSF MMPs, reflecting extracellular matrix breakdown; CSF neurofilament, a marker of axonal damage; and blood inflammatory cytokines and adhesion molecules, were identified. The investigators suggested that the profile of SSVD biomarkers contrasted with the characteristic CSF profile of AD (ie, Aβ peptide and increased phosphorylated and total tau [t-tau]).[9] One should keep in mind that neuropathological findings of AD and cerebrovascular disease frequently coexist in older community populations, and thus, one may anticipate a mixed picture of cerebrovascular and neurodegenerative biomarkers.

In a review by Hosoki and colleagues,[10] similarities between biomarkers in acute ischemic stroke and vascular dementia were discussed. Biomarkers of oxidative stress, endothelial dysfunction, inflammation, and neuronal injury were emphasized.[10] Also, there was mention of the importance of identification of reliable markers of brain tissue damage, microRNAs, and long noncoding RNAs. MicroRNAs may be of relevance mechanistically as regulators of function of the blood–brain barrier, influencers of apoptosis and oxidative stress, and modulators of neuroinflammation. In another review on emerging biomarkers in VCI and dementia, Cipollini and colleagues[11] discussed the pathophysiology of endothelial dysfunction, blood–brain barrier disruption, and neuroinflammation, and in addition reference biomarkers of coagulation and thrombosis, and circulating microRNAs.

Vascular contributions to cognitive impairment are likely to be an important factor in the pathogenesis of cognitive impairment.[12] Studies have shown that early and midlife cardiovascular risk factors are associated with subsequent cognitive impairment, and the trajectory of cognitive decline and incident dementia is related to an accelerated trajectory of cardiovascular risks.[1,13] Furthermore, the aforementioned reviews of VCI[9–11] support a mechanistic landscape of underlying factors such as oxidative stress, endothelial dysfunction, neuroinflammation, and extracellular matrix breakdown. What has been lacking, however, is a large scale, comprehensive, translational study of VCI biomarker candidates. To answer this question an initiative on vascular contributions to cognitive impairment, MARKVCID (Biomarkers for Vascular Contributions to Cognitive Impairment and Dementia Consortium) has been established and is discussed below.[14]

MARKVCID includes seven original research sites and a coordinating center funded by grants from the US National Institute of Neurological Disorders and Stroke, National Institute on Aging, and BrightFocus Foundation.[14] The initiative is largely focused on SSVD, the most common phenotype of VCI. The initial 5-year mission of the study is to analyze and optimize candidate VCI and dementia biomarkers in years 1 to 2 and develop and carryout a biomarker scaling up, multisite protocol and validation in years 3 to 5.[14] To achieve the goals of the study, the following protocols or procedures have been established: clinical/cognitive measure collection manuals; biospecimen collection best practices; imaging standard operating procedures; patient MRI protocols; phantom MRI protocols; imaging-based biomarker kit protocols; and fluid-based biomarker kit protocols.[14]

The primary focus of the study is identification of brain imaging and blood and CSF biomarkers. For example, the first phase of the study focused on but was not limited to the following imaging biomarkers: MRI FLAIR, diffusion, gradient echo, T2-weighted imaging, and cerebrovascular reactivity to better understand brain white matter volume, progression or regression, and blood vessel stiffness leading to impairment of cerebral autoregulation and perfusion.[14] In relation to blood and CSF biomarkers, the first phase of the study focused on the following fluid biomarkers: (1) angiogenic factors (factors that regulate the growth and development of blood vessels; eg, vascular endothelial growth factor); (2) cytokines (mediators of inflammation; eg, interleukins 6 and 8); and (3) proteases (eg, MMPs). Based on the results of the first phase of human study, the second phase of the study is moving forward with further testing. The MARKVCID Web site includes links to the publications that have come forth from the study thus far, much of which has informed the second phase of the study, but as of yet, the results are not definitive in relation to clinical practice.[14]

Overall and based on MARKVCID findings thus far, biomarker identification for VCI remains a work in progress with promising leads to inform the way forward in relation to potential mechanisms and pathways whereby interventions may be developed to prevent or slow cognitive impairment associated with cerebrovascular disease. We now transition to the status of biomarkers in AD, an area of study that is more advanced in comparison to that for VCI.

KEY BIOMARKERS IN ALZHEIMER'S DISEASE

There have been many recent advances in the discovery and development of biomarkers for AD. Such measures focus on key neuropathological manifestations of AD such as Aβ plaques, tau neurofibrillary tangles (NFTs), and neurodegeneration.[15] Beyond structural changes of the brain in cognitively impairing disorders that may be detected by commercial CT and MRI of the brain, neuroimaging advances such as amyloid-PET, tau-PET, and fluorodeoxyglucose-PET scans are also now available in some regions.[16] However, neuroimaging poses challenges in relation to availability, cost, and tolerance to the procedure. Thus, there has been interest in the development of blood and CSF biomarkers for AD, as these studies, especially when blood based, provide an easy route of access and a potentially more affordable option.[17] The author now explores candidate biomarker tests for AD to provide a simple understanding of the potential role for these tests.

Before one considers candidate biomarkers, a brief review of the neuropathological staging of AD is provided. As mentioned in Rupal I. Mehta and Julie A. Schneider's article, "Neuropathology of the Common Forms of Dementia," in this issue, two of the hallmarks of AD neuropathology are deposition of the abnormal proteins, Aβ in the form of extracellular plaques, and irregularly phosphorylated forms of the microtubule-associated protein tau, manifesting as intraneuronal NFTs. Aβ plaques precede the appearance of NFTs in the brain.[17] Initially, NFTs are found in the trans-entorhinal cortex, near to the entorhinal cortex. As disease progresses, NFTs involve the entorhinal cortex, an area that connects the hippocampus to main portions of the cerebral cortex (neocortex), and the hippocampus and neocortical brain regions become involved. Tau may be important in relation to symptoms of AD, as the presence of tau, neurodegeneration, or both may be needed for memory decline to occur, whereas this is not the case for Aβ.[18] It has been argued, however, that amyloid pathology may provide a permissive state or acts as an enabler whereby tau-related hippocampal brain dysfunction may occur.[19] In relation to the deposition of Aβ in the brain, initially it is deposited within the neocortex followed by spread into areas such as the entorhinal cortex and hippocampus and later into subcortical nuclei including the basal ganglia, thalamus, and hypothalamus, and eventually into the brainstem and cerebellum.

Importantly, as AD brain changes progress, the CSF, which serves as a draining system for Aβ outflow from the central nervous system, shows less Aβ, whereas t-tau and p-tau, the major component of NFTs in the brain and a marker of neuronal injury and neurodegeneration, are elevated in the CSF.

Based on the scope of this brief review, select AD biomarkers and studies are discussed below to provide key teaching points.

- *Amyloid Beta*: Aβ may be measured in the plasma or CSF. The ratio of Aβ 42 (the main component of amyloid plaques in the brain) to Aβ 40 has evolved as a useful biomarker of cognitive impairment. For example, in the Atherosclerosis Risk in Communities cohort, the Aβ 42: Aβ 40 plasma ratio was predictive of a 37% reduction in the risk of mild cognitive impairment (MCI) or dementia in later life compared with a 13% reduction with Aβ 42 alone and a 15% increase with Aβ 40 alone.[20] In a head-to-head comparison of different plasma Aβ 42: Aβ 40 assays in AD, mass spectrometry was shown to be the technology of choice.[21] In the CSF, data suggest that Aβ 42: Aβ 40 is also favored over Aβ 42 alone as there is a higher correlation with tau markers.[22]

- *Tau*: Tau may be measured in the plasma or CSF in a number of different forms: t-tau and p-tau with the latter form being the major component of NFTs in the brain.[17] p-tau consists of various subtypes (eg, p-tau231, p-tau217, p-tau181). In the Presymptomatic Evaluation of Experimental or Novel Treatments for Alzheimer Disease cohort, plasma p-tau231 was more strongly linked to PET biomarkers of AD than p-tau181, and the combination of p-tau and Aβ 42: Aβ 40 biomarkers preferentially detected early AD pathologic change and cognitive decline.[23] In addition, in the AD Neuroimaging Initiative, CSF t-tau, and p-tau181 discriminated between autopsy-confirmed AD and other dementias.[24]

- *Neurofilament Light and Glial Acidic Fibrillary Protein*: Plasma neurofilament light chain (NfL) is a protein and general marker of neurodegeneration. As such, it is not specific for AD.[25] Glial acidic fibrillary protein (GFAP) is a marker of astrogliosis (astrocytic activation) or glial–astrocytic injury which increases when there is Aβ pathology or other neurodegenerative brain change, and thus, is not a specific biomarker for AD.[25] NfL may be associated with worse white matter disease of the brain based on cross-sectional data.[26] In addition, NfL and GFAP in combination have been used in studies to predict risk of AD or other cognitive decline and have generally been shown to be useful biomarkers.[27–29]

Box 1 shows the AD biomarkers that have been approved by the US federal drug administration (FDA) for commercial use as well as additional biomarker tests that are available. The biomarkers are grouped according to neuroimaging and fluid categories and are accompanied by a brief description of their indication.

Box 1
US FDA approved neuroimaging and fluid biomarkers available for the diagnosis of Alzheimer's disease and other causes of cognitive impairment[a]

Neuroimaging Biomarkers
1. *Florbetapir F 18 Injection* (Amyvid): Radioactive diagnostic agent for PET imaging of the brain to determine β-amyloid neuritic plaque density in adults with cognitive impairment who are being evaluated for Alzheimer's disease (AD) or other causes of cognitive decline. Reference Source: https://www.accessdata.fda.gov/drugsatfda_docs/nda/2012/202008Orig1s000Approv.pdf (accessed online July 14, 2022).
2. *Flutemetamol F 18 injection* (Vizamyl): Radioactive diagnostic agent for PET imaging of the brain with a similar indication to #1 above. Reference Source: https://www.accessdata.fda.gov/drugsatfda_docs/nda/2013/203137Orig1s000Approv.pdf (accessed online July 14, 2022)
3. *Florbetaben F18 injection* (Neuraceq): Radioactive diagnostic agent for PET imaging of the brain with a similar indication to #1 above. Reference Source: https://www.accessdata.fda.gov/drugsatfda_docs/nda/2014/204677Orig1s000Approv.pdf (accessed online July 14, 2022).
4. *Flortaucipir F18 injection* (Tauvid): Radioactive diagnostic agent indicated for PET imaging of the brain to determine the density and distribution of aggregated tau neurofibrillary tangles (NFTs) in adult patients with cognitive impairment who are being evaluated for AD. Reference Source: https://www.accessdata.fda.gov/drugsatfda_docs/nda/2020/212123Orig1s000Approv.pdf (accessed online July 14, 2022)

Fluid Biomarkers
5. *β-Amyloid Ratio (1–42/1–40)* (Lumipulse G): Cerebrospinal fluid (CSF) test that combines the results of Lumipulse G P-Amyloid 1-42 and Lumipulse G P-Amyloid 1-40 assays into a ratio of B-amyloid 1_42 to B-amyloid 1_40 concentrations using the LUMIPULSE G 1200 System to be used in adult patients, aged 55 years and older, presenting with cognitive impairment who are being evaluated for AD or other causes of cognitive decline. Reference Source: https://www.accessdata.fda.gov/cdrh_docs/reviews/DEN200072.pdf (accessed online July 14, 2022)
6. *Phosphorylated Tau (pTau) 181 Protein and Apolipoprotein (APOE) E4 (Elecsys Amyloid Plasma Panel)*: Measures blood plasma pTau and APOE E4 and is used in conjunction with other clinical information in symptomatic patients who are being evaluated for AD and other causes of cognitive decline to ensure better identification of patients that require further confirmatory testing. The test received US FDA Breakthrough Device Designation as did the Elecsys Beta Amyloid (1–42) CSF and Elecsys Phospho-Tau (181P) CSF tests. Reference Source: www.roche.com (accessed online July 24, 2022)

[a]Additional tests available to measure biomarkers in AD: A. *Amyloid-beta 42:40 levels and ApoE Isoforms* (PrecivityAD): Amyloid-beta mass spectrometry assay used to monitor amyloid-beta 42:40 levels and ApoE isoforms in the blood. Reference Source: https://precivityad.com/ (accessed online July 15, 2022). B. *Amyloid-beta 42:40 levels* (AD-Detect): Amyloid-beta mass spectrometry assay used to monitor amyloid-beta 42:40 levels in the blood. Reference Source: https://testdirectory.questdiagnostics.com/test/test-guides/TS_AD_Detect_BetaRatioPlasma/quest-ad-detect (accessed online July 15, 2022). C. *Neurofilament Light Chain:* Blood test to assess neuronal damage related to various neurodegenerative diseases. Reference Source: https://www.labcorp.com/tests/140455/neurofilament-light-chain-serum (accessed online, July 15, 2022).

A number of other approaches are being studied in relation to biomarkers for cognitively impairing disorders, and a detailed discussion of these approaches is outside the scope of this article. For example, genomic exploration is being carried out to elucidate genomic susceptibility profiles for cognitive dysfunction.[30] As an example, there are a number of genetic mutations associated with amyloid precursor protein, a potential biomarker target for intervention to reduce Aβ burden in the brain. Furthermore, the presence of an APOE epsilon 4 allele substantially elevates the risk of AD and may be used as a marker to select those persons more likely to have AD changes in the brain and who may be candidates for AD interventions. In addition, epigenetic approaches are being explored to better understand how behavior and environment alter how genes work through methylation of DNA whereby genes are "turned off" and through demethylation of DNA whereby genes are "turned on" to function. In one study, DNA methylation metrics were associated with MRI markers of brain aging whereby blood C-reactive protein was not.[31] Genome-wide association studies and genetic molecular characterization of vascular and perivascular cells in AD support a mechanistic vascular pathological underpinning in AD.[32,33] Finally, digital technology is being applied to AD whereby voice recordings may be used to identify persons with cognitive impairment.[34]

POTENTIAL LIMITATIONS OF BIOMARKERS AND APPLICATION IN CLINICAL PRACTICE

In response to the publication reframing the definition of AD based on a biological construct and reliance on biomarkers,[4] an expert panel published a personal view on the limitations of biomarkers and how they may be applied in a clinical setting.[35] When considering a pure biological definition and relying on biomarkers in AD, the investigators highlight specific limitations that one must bear in mind. These include distinction between the presence of AD neuropathology and the complete AD continuum of phenotypic clinical features plus neuropathology; the potential for a low predictive accuracy of biomarkers in AD (eg, in MCI); the co-occurrence of other neuropathological processes in AD patients (eg, Lewy body disease or cerebrovascular disease) which need to be recognized for prognostic and management considerations but may be overlooked; variability in the prognostic value of biomarkers in relation to, for example, cognitive decline; limits of generalizability and accessibility of biomarkers; and other pertinent limitations.[35]

From an application in clinical practice perspective, the panel makes the following key points to inform the health care practitioner about how to apply AD biomarkers in practice[35]:

1. Consider AD as a continuum including its clinical phenotype (ie, signs and symptoms such as amnestic manifestations) and biomarker measures.
2. In persons with common phenotypic manifestations of AD (eg, amnestic syndrome), positivity of Aβ and tau biomarkers establishes a diagnosis.
3. Recommended biomarkers: low CSF Aβ 42, increased CSF Aβ 40-42 ratio (preferable to low CSF Aβ) or high tracer retention for amyloid-PET. For tau, high CSF p-tau or increased ligand retention for tau-PET. If the results of cognitive, biomarker or both tests are of borderline significance, additional investigations may be needed (eg, repeat testing, fluorodeoxyglucose-PET).
4. CSF testing may be preferable for some patients to obtain simultaneous Aβ and tau measure.
5. In routine clinical practice, AD biomarkers are generally not indicated in cognitively unimpaired persons based on the inability of these metrics to predict cognitive trajectories in asymptomatic persons.

6. Biomarker positivity may be ambiguous in cases of concurrent (mixed) neuropathology.
7. Biomarker investigations may be used for screening purposes for interventional and other research studies.
8. It may be propitious to have AD biomarkers selected, ordered, and interpreted by health care providers with special expertise in the field.

In relation to tau biomarkers in AD, a recently published expert review states that only 5% to 10% of Aβ-positive cognitively unimpaired persons and 50% to 67% of Aβ-positive persons with MCI have suprathreshold tau-PET signal in the neocortex, whereas both CSF and plasma p-tau markers may be elevated in early disease stages.[17] However, given key limitations in CSF and fluid tau biomarkers, tau-PET may be the preferred initial biomarker test for the differential diagnosis of dementia syndromes.[17]

CLINICS CARE POINTS

- Biomarkers should be interpreted within the context of the clinical phenotype of the underlying dementia subtype.
- As the Alzheimer's disease (AD) process progresses in the brain, amyloid beta (Aβ) levels drop, and measures of tau increase in the cerebrospinal fluid (CSF).
- A useful biomarker in the CSF and blood is the ratio of Aβ 42: Aβ 40.
- The value of AD biomarkers in asymptomatic persons remains uncertain, is primarily a research tool, and may best be interpreted by persons with special expertise in the field.
- Biomarkers for vascular cognitive impairment are currently under study and are not ready for application in clinical practice.

DISCLOSURE

Dr P.B. Gorelick serves on a Data and Safety Monitoring Board for Novartis in relation to a heart failure and cognition study.

REFERENCES

1. Gorelick PB, Furie K, Iadecola C, et al. Defining optimal brain health in adults: a presidential advisory from the American Heart Association/American Stroke Association. Stroke 2017;48:e284–303.
2. Hachinski V, Einhaupt K, Ganten D, et al. Preventing dementia by preventing stroke: the Berlin Manifesto. Alzheimer's Dement 2019;15(7):961–84.
3. Sweeney MD, Mantagne A, Sagre AP, et al. Vascular dysfunction—the disregarded partner of Alzheimer's disease. Alzheimer's Demen 2019;15:158–67.
4. Jack CR Jr, Bennett DA, Blennow K, et al. NIA-AA research framework: toward a biological definition of Alzheimer's disease. Alzheimer's Demen 2018;14:535–62.
5. Amur A, FDA-NIH Biomarker Working Group. Available at: https://www.ncbi.nlm.nih.gov/books/NBK326791/. Accessed online, March 2022.
6. Gorelick PB. Vascular cognitive impairment (Chapter 6). In: Lazar RM, Pavol MA, Browndyke JN, editors. Neurovascular neuropsychology. 2nd edition. Cham, Switzerland: Springer; 2020. p. 121–38.
7. Rosenberg GA, Kornfeld M, Storving J, et al. Subcortical arteriosclerotic encephalopathy (Binswanger): computerized tomography. Neurology 1979;29(8):1102–6.

8. Rosenberg GA. Matrix metalloproteinase-mediated neuroinflammation in vascular cognitive impairment of the binswanger type. Cell Mol Neurobiol 2016; 36(2):195–202.
9. Wallin A, Kapaki E, Boban M, et al. Biochemical markers in vascular cognitive impairment associated with subcortical small vessel disease - a consensus report. BMC Neurol 2017;17. Article number: 102.
10. Hosoki S, Tanaka T, Ihara M. Diagnostic and prognostic blood biomarkers in vascular dementia: from the viewpoint of ischemic stroke. Neurochem Int 2021; 146:105015.
11. Cipollini V, Trolli F, Giubilei F. Emerging biomarkers in vascular cognitive impairment and dementia: from pathophysiological pathways to clinical application. Int J Mol Sci 2019;20:2812.
12. Gorelick PB, Scuteri A, Black SE, et al. Vascular contributions to cognitive impairment and dementia. Stroke 2011;42:2672–713.
13. Von Cederwald BF, Josefsson M, Wahlin A, et al. Association of cardiovascular risk trajectory with cognitive decline and incident dementia. Neurology 2022; 98:e2013–22.
14. MARKVCID website. Available at: https://markvcid.partners.org/about/consortium-overview. Accessed July 12, 2022.
15. Grill JD, Karlawish J. Disclosing Alzheimer disease biomarker results to research participants. JAMA Neurol 2022;79:645–6.
16. Scheltens P, De Strooper B, Kivipelto M, et al. Alzheimer's disease. Lancet 2021; 397:1577–90.
17. Ossenkoppele R, van der Kant R, Hansson O. Tau biomarkers in Alzheimer's disease: toward implementation in clinical practice and trials. Lancet Neurol 2022; 21:726–34.
18. Jack CR Jr, Wiste HJ, Therneau TM, et al. Associations of amyloid, tau, and neurodegeneration biomarker profiles with rates of memory decline among individuals without dementia. JAMA 2019;321(23):2316–25.
19. Duzel E, Ziegler G, Berron D, et al. Amyloid pathology but not APOE e4status is permissive for tau-related hippocampal dysfunction. Brain 2022;145:1473–85.
20. Sullivan KJ, Blackshear C, Simino J, et al. Association of midlife plasma amyloid-beta levels with cognitive impairment in late life. Neurology 2021;97:e1123–31.
21. Janelidze S, Teunlssen CE, Zetterberg H, et al. Head-to-head comparison of 8 plasma amyloid-beta 42/40 assays in Alzheimer's disease. JAMA Neurol 2021; 78(11):1375–82.
22. Delaby C, Estelles T, Zhu N, et al. Alzheimer's Res Ther 2022;14:20. https://doi.org/10.1186/s13195-022-00967-z.
23. Meyer P-F, Ashton N-J, Karikari T-K, et al. Plasma p-tau231, p-tau 181, PET biomarkers, and cognitive change in older adults. Ann Neurol 2022;91:548–60.
24. Grothe MJ, Moscoso A, Ashton NJ, et al. Associations of fully automated CSF and novel plasma biomarkers with Alzheimer's disease neuropathology at autopsy. Neurology 2021;97:e1229–42.
25. Head E, Zetterberg H. Commentary on Oeckl et al., "Serum Beta-Synuclein is Higher in Down's Syndrome and Precedes Rise of pTau181". Ann Neurol 2022; 92:3–5.
26. Fohner AE, Bartz TM, Tracy RP, et al. Association of serum neurofilament light chain concentration and MRI findings in older adults. The Cardiovascular Health Study. Neurology 2022;98:e903–11.
27. Schindler SE, Bateman RJ. Combining blood-based biomarkers to predict risk for Alzheimer's disease dementia. Nat Aging 2021;1:26–8.

28. Ebernau JL, Pelkmans W, Verberk IMW, et al. Association of CSF, plasma, and imaging markers of neurodegeneration with clinical progression in people with subjective cognitive impairment. Neurology 2022;98:e1315–26.

29. Stevenson-Hoare J, Heslegrave A, Leonenko G, et al. Plasma biomarkers and genetics in the diagnosis and prediction of Alzheimer's disease. Brain 2022;awac128. https://doi.org/10.1093/brain/awac128. Online ahead of print.

30. Caselli RJ, Beach TG, Knopman DS, et al. Alzheimer's disease: scientific breakthroughs and translational challenges. Mayo Clin Proc 2017;92(6):978–94.

31. Conole ELS, Stevenson AJ, Maniega SM, et al. DNA methylation and protein markers of chronic inflammation and their associations with brain and cognitive aging. Neurology 2021;97:e2340–52.

32. Bellenguez C, Kucukali F, Jansen IE, et al. New insights into the genetic etiology of Alzheimer's disease and related dementias. Nat Genet 2022;54:412–36.

33. Yang AC, Vest RT, Kern F, et al. A human brain vascular atlas reveals diverse mediators of Alzheimer's risk. Nature 2022;603:885–92.

34. Amini S, Hao B, Zhang L, et al. Automated detection of mild cognitive impairment and dementia from voice recordings: a natural language processing approach. Alzheimer's Dement 2022;1–10. https://doi.org/10.1002/alz.12721.

35. Dubois B, Villain N, Frisoni GB, et al. Clinical diagnosis of Alzheimer's disease: recommendations of the international working group. Lancet Neurol 2021;20: 484–96.

What Are the Key Diagnostic Cognitive Impairment and Dementia Subtypes and How to Integrate all of the Diagnostic Data to Establish a Diagnosis?

Sheena Baratono, MD PhD, Daniel Press, MD*

KEYWORDS

- Mild cognitive impairment • Alzheimer's disease • Lewy body dementia
- Frontotemporal dementia • Vascular dementia
- Limbic-predominant age-related TDP-43 encephalopathy
- Primary progressive aphasia

KEY POINTS

- Progression of mild cognitive impairment to dementia occurs with loss of activities of daily function.
- Memory loss is a common complaint for a variety of dementias beyond Alzheimer's disease and amnestic mild cognitive impairment (MCI).
- Early memory loss and rapid forgetting is a hallmark of typical Alzheimer's disease.
- Visual hallucinations and parkinsonism are commonly seen in Lewy body disease.
- Behavioral changes are common in behavioral variant frontotemporal dementia, whereas language issues are seen in the primary progressive aphasias.
- Small-vessel ischemic changes are seen in imaging in vascular dementia.
- Mixed dementia phenotypes are common.

INTRODUCTION

In this issue, neuropsychological screening and formal testing (David L. Nyenhuis and Jaclyn Reckow's article, "Office- and Bedside-Based Screening for Cognitive Impairment and the Dementias: Which Tools to Use, Interpreting the Results and What Are the Next Steps?"; and Victor A. Del Bene and colleagues' article, "Formal Neuropsychological Testing: Test Batteries, Interpretation, and Added Value in

Cognitive Neurology Unit, Beth Israel Deaconess Medical Center, 330 Brookline Avenue, Brookline, MA 02215, USA
* Corresponding author.
E-mail address: dpress@bidmc.harvard.edu

Clin Geriatr Med 39 (2023) 77–90
https://doi.org/10.1016/j.cger.2022.08.002
0749-0690/23/© 2022 Elsevier Inc. All rights reserved.
geriatric.theclinics.com

Practice," in this issue), neuroimaging (Borna Bonakdarpour and Clara Takarabe's article, "Brain Networks, Clinical Manifestations, and Neuroimaging: The Role of CT, MRI, PET and Other Advanced Neuroimaging Tests," in this issue), and blood and cerebrospinal fluid markers (Philip B. Gorelick's article, "Blood and Cerebrospinal Fluid Biomarkers in Vascular Dementia and Alzheimer's Disease: A Brief Review," in this issue) have previously been reviewed. We now focus on how to integrate this information into the clinic when evaluating a patient. First, we will discsus staging the severity of the deficit, for instance, mild cognitive impairment versus dementia. Next, we will focus on determining the clinical syndrome and underlying pathology. After the introductory remarks that include diagnostic guides for distinguishing broad and more specific categories of cognitive impairment, we follow a case-based approach to establish a diagnosis of common causes of cognitive impairment according to patient complaints and common presentations.

The most common complaint patients report is memory loss, which is often vague. It can refer to a variety of cognitive abnormalities including true amnesia but also word finding difficulties, difficulty with concentration and attention, or depression and anxiety. The most common memory complaint seen with typical Alzheimer's disease (AD) is rapid forgetting but patients can present with false memories or distortions as well.[1] A patient's insight into their memory deficits is highly variable, making information from a caregiver or other informant critical for an accurate history. We recommend following a core diagnostic evaluation including a history, physical examination, cognitive testing, and imaging. Questions that are helpful when differentiating normal aging from pathologic cognitive decline include changes in the patient's judgment, less interest in hobbies or activities, repeating the same questions or stories, trouble learning how to use new technology or tools, impairment of orientation to time, difficulty managing finances, difficulty remembering appointments, and daily problems with memory or thinking.[2]

Staging a patient's memory deficits from subjective memory concerns to mild cognitive impairment to dementia is important for diagnosis, prognosis, treatment, and care planning. Subjective memory concerns becomes mild cognitive impairment when there is objective measurement of decline in one or more cognitive domains.[3] The transition to dementia is denoted by the loss of the patient's ability to largely maintain their instrumental activities of daily living such as managing finances, cooking, and transportation[3–5] (**Box 1**). Age of onset of symptoms is also important. Early-onset AD begins before age 65 and accounts for 5% to 6% of cases of AD.[6] Approximately 11% of patients with early-onset AD have familial AD with a mutation in presenilin 1 or 2 or amyloid precursor protein.[6] Any patient with a family history of early-onset AD should be counseled about the availability of genetic testing for these mutations. The APOE4/E4 genotype is the most substantial genetic risk factor for late-onset AD and testing can aid diagnosis and prognosis in patients with a family history of late-onset AD.[1] Frontotemporal dementia begins as early as the fourth decade of life and peaks in the 5th and 6th decade, accounting for a large percentage of early-onset dementias. Lewy body dementia and vascular dementia show less of an age predilection.

Important questions to ask regarding a patient's cognitive status include short-term memory such as rapidly forgetting information, repeating themselves, or misplacing objects. It is very important to assess whether these memory impairments were the first noticeable symptoms and whether they are the dominant symptoms over time. Memory predominant neurodegenerative causes of dementia include AD, which is the most common, but also limbic-predominant age-related TAR DNA-binding protein-43 (TDP-43) encephalopathy. The two are difficult to tell apart clinically but limbic-predominant age-related TDP-43 encephalopathy shows relatively isolated hippocampal atrophy on structural imaging and is negative for amyloid and tau on

---

Box 1
Instrumental activities of daily living

The Functional Assessment Questionnaire assesses instrumental activities of daily living. Evaluation should take into account a patient's baseline functional capacity and any subsequent changes.

Examples of instrumental activities of daily living:
• Writing checks and maintaining other financial resources.
• Assembling tax or business records.
• Shopping alone for clothes, household necessities, or groceries.
• Playing a game of skill or working on a hobby.
• Heating foods on the stove, making a cup of coffee, and turning the stove off.
• Preparing a well-balanced meal.
• Keeping track of current events.
• Paying attention to, understanding, and discussing TV, books, or movies.
• Remembering appointments, family occasions, holidays, and medications.
• Traveling out of the neighborhood, driving, arranging to take public transportation.

Data from Refs.[20–22]

---

biomarker testing.[7] Limbic-predominant age-related TDP-43 occurs mostly in patients in their 80s to 90s.[7]

Language difficulties are also common chief complaints presented most often as word-finding difficulties. It is helpful to evaluate whether the word-finding is the predominant symptom as both AD and frontotemporal dementia can present with primary progressive aphasia phenotypes. Logopenic primary progressive aphasia is usually caused by Alzheimer's pathology and causes difficulties with word finding and repetition, similar to a conduction aphasia. They often use platitudes and are described as having "empty speech" which has low meaningful content. Semantic and nonfluent/agramamtic variant primary progressive aphasias are usually a frontotemporal dementia caused by TDP-43 or tau. Semantic variant primary progressive aphasia patients' word-finding difficulties are associated with impaired conceptual understanding of words, anomia, poor object knowledge, and paraphasic errors. It is similar to Wernicke's aphasia. Nonfluent/agrammatic primary progressive aphasia is notable for having agrammatic and effortful speech and is more similar to a Broca's aphasia.

Changes in behavior and a loss of empathy are important early signs of behavioral variant frontotemporal dementia. These patients can also present with executive dysfunction including trouble with sequencing, perseveration and may have frontal release signs on exam. Visual hallucinations, changes in autonomic function, REM behavior sleep disorder, and parkinsonism are the hallmarks of Lewy body dementia. Lastly, it is important to assess for vascular risk factors as vascular cognitive impairment is common and potentially modifiable or preventable (**Table 1**). Ref 22 Keep in mind that patients may present with a mixture of symptoms and underlying pathologies.

The physical examination is a critical component when diagnosing dementia. It should include evaluation for parkinsonism, particularly if Lewy body dementia is a concern. Parkinsonism findings include shuffling of gait, bradykinesia, resting tremor, and rigidity. Frontal release signs can be useful when frontotemporal dementia is a possible diagnosis. Frontal release signs include the snout, suck, glabellar and palmomental reflexes.[8] Bloodwork can be helpful when the presentation is vague such as when a patient presents with encephalopathy or delirium and to rule out nondegenerative causes of cognitive impairment including memory loss. Tests include Vitamin B12, thyroid stimulating hormone (TSH), and basic tests such as a compelte blood count and comprehensive metabolic panel to evaluate for metabolic disease or

Table 1
Pathologies and prominent features

Disease	Pathology	Prominent Feature	Prevalence
Alzheimer's disease	Amyloid beta, Tau	Memory loss	~75%
Vascular disease	Small vessel ischemic disease, stroke	Executive dysfunction	~15%–25%
Limbic predominate age-related TDP-43 encephalopathy	TDP-43	Memory loss	~10%–20%
Lewy body disease	Alpha-synuclein	Visual hallucinations, Parkinsonism	~10%–15%
Frontal temporal dementia	Tau or TDP-43	Executive dysfunction, personality changes	~5%

Data from Budson AE, Solomon PR. Chapter 2 - Evaluating the Patient with Memory Loss or Dementia. In: Hudson AE, Solomon PR, eds. Memory Loss, Alzheimer's Disease, and Dementia (Second Edition). Elsevier; 2016:5-38. https://doi.org/10.1016/B978-0-323-28661-9.00002-0.

infection. Vitamin B12 deficiency is common in the elderly, often due to loss of intrinsic factors leading to decreased absorption of Vitamin B12. Such deficiency can lead to multiple neurologic symptoms including hyperreflexia and neuropathy as well as altered mood and cognition.[9] Thyroid dysfunction, particularly hypothyroidism, can cause impaired memory and slowed cognition as well as mood instability or depression.[10] The time course of the symptoms is also extremely helpful in diagnosis, with an insidious onset and gradual progression suggesting a neurodegenerative disorder, an acute onset or stepwise decline suggesting a vascular etiology, and rapid onset with inattention raising concern for a toxic-metabolic process, neoplasm, autoimmune disease, infectious process, or prion disease.[11]

Brain imaging should be done in all patients with cognitive decline, with brain MRI being the preferred modality to evaluate for atrophy as well as inflammation, neoplasm, or other relevant pathology. If an MRI is unobtainable, computed tomography (CT) of the brain can be used in its place; however, there may be a poorer resolution of atrophy, inflamamtion and vascular burden.[12] Notably, brain MRI but not CT can identify old bleeds as seen in cerebral amyloid angiopathy which can be present in AD.[13] When trying to discern whether a patient has frontotemporal dementia versus Lewy body dementia or AD, an flu-deoxyglucose (FDG)-PET or single-photon emission computed tomography (SPECT) can be helpful.[1,8,14] Both of these tests identify brain regions with reduced activity or decreased metabolism suggesting that they are damaged. Biomarker testing can also be useful but is currently limited in availability. A lumbar puncture and cerebral spinal fluid (CSF) analysis for amyloid beta and tau ratios has high sensitivity and specificity in AD and is particularly beneficial in young onset AD or in atypical presentations.[1] In addition, a patient's "amyloid status" can also be assessed either by amyloid PET studies or with serum amyloid-beta tests, though access to both tests is limited.[1] Specific tests to detect Lewy body dementia include an in-lab sleep study to evaluate for REM behavior sleep disorder and dopamine imaging. More recently, confirmation of pathologic alpha-synuclein can be verified by skin biopsy.[15] See **Box 2** for diagnostic criteria including more indicative imaging studies for diagnosis of the dementias.

Cognitive testing includes bedside screening tests and detailed testing done by neuropsychology specialists. Comprehensive neuropsychological testing provides a full neurocognitive profile and can provide guidance on how to maximize cognitive

---

Box 2
Diagnostic parameters for dementias

- Lewy body dementia[19]
  - Essential: Progressive cognitive impairment leading to impairment in activities of daily living.
    - Cognitive impairment can vary and include impaired executive function, attention, visuospatial processing, and memory impairment.
  - Core criteria:
  - Recurrent visual hallucinations that are well formed.
  - REM behavior sleep disorder
  - Parkinsonism including bradykinesia, rigidity, or rest tremor.
  - Fluctuations in cognition, attention, or alertness.

- Supportive features:
  - Autonomic dysfunction including postural instability, orthostasis, constipation, or incontinence.
  - Decreased sense of smell.
  - Severe sensitivity to anti-psychotics, particularly typical antipsychotics.
  - Hypersomnia.
  - Postural instability.
  - Psychiatric comorbidities.
  - Repeated falls.
  - Non-visual hallucinations

- Biomarkers:
  - Reduced basal ganglia dopamine uptake on SPECT or PET.
  - Low uptake on iodine 123-MIBG myocardial scintigraphy.
  - Confirmation of REM sleep behavior disorder.
  - More recently, skin biopsy for alpha-synuclein has been shown to be sensitive for the diagnosis of Lewy body dementia but was not established when the last consensus criteria were established in 2017.[15]

- Exclusion: Presentation cannot be better explained by another diagnosis.
  - Parkinson's disease with dementia can be difficult to tell apart from Lewy body dementia but patients present first with parkinsonism and then develop other hallmarks of Lewy body disease.

- Alzheimer's disease[3]
- Dementia is defined as progressive objective cognitive impairment leading to impairment in activities of daily living.
  - Insidious onset.
    - Clear worsening in cognition.
    - Initial and clearest cognitive deficits are related to:
    - Memory
    - Word finding
    - Visuospatial processing
    - Executive dysfunction.
    - Presentation cannot be better explained by another diagnosis.

- Behavioral variant frontotemporal dementia23
  - Required: Progressive deterioration of behavior and/or cognition.
  - 3 of 6:
    - Disinhibition (inappropriate behavior)
    - Apathy or inertia
    - Loss of sympathy or empathy
    - Perseverative, ritualistic or stereotyped behaviors
    - Hyperorality or dietary changes
    - Executive dysfunction on testing with relative sparing of memory and visuospatial functioning.
- Imaging supportive findings:
  - Frontal temporal atrophy on structural CT or MRI or hypometabolism on SPECT or FDG-PET.

○ Exclusion: cannot be better explained by another medical or neurodegenerative process.
- Vascular-dementia[5]
- DSM V criteria for vascular cognitive impairment:
  ▪ Onset of symptoms correlates with cerebrovascular events.
  ▪ Executive function and attention decline are prominent.
  ▪ There is evidence of cerebrovascular disease based on history, examination and/or neuroimaging.

reserve and function. Formal neuropsychological testing is particularly useful when there is diagnostic uncertainty and in early-onset patients (see **Box 2**).

CASE 1: MILD COGNITIVE IMPAIRMENT: AMNESTIC

- Chief complaint: "I'm having trouble remembering."
- History:
- A 74-year-old woman with hypertension and hyperlipidemia presents with short-term memory loss and difficulty multitasking. She reports that she is not remembering recent conversations or events as well as she used to. She was running a small company until a few years ago but stopped after noting trouble multitasking and organizing work tasks. She has been under significant stress after a family member was diagnosed with breast cancer and she has minor depression and anxiety. Her husband reports that she still manages the finances, has not made any errors, but she will have him check them more often than she used to. She does not smoke and drinks alcohol only on special occasions. She has trouble falling and staying asleep. Her husband notes she does not snore nor move in her sleep.
  ○ Family history: Both parents developed dementia in their late 80s. She thinks her father had AD, but her mother was thought to have vascular dementia.
  ○ Activities of daily living: She has not made any mistakes cooking or driving. She follows current events and continues her hobbies of knitting and reading without difficulty. She is not making mistakes when shopping and uses a shopping list. She does not miss doses of her medications or appointments.
- Physical examination: There is no evidence of parkinsonism on movement or gait testing.
- Cognitive testing: 24/30 on the montreal cognitive assessment (MoCA). She missed points for the cube copy, fluency, and 1/5 on delayed recall, getting two of the missed items correct with multiple choice but two items are lost.
- Imaging testing: A structural MRI without contrast showed mild global volume loss without disproportional hippocampal volume loss and mild angiopathic changes thought to be small vessel ischemic disease.
- Ancillary testing
  ○ Neuropsychological testing: Given her mix of memory and executive dysfunction complaints, full neuropsychological testing was performed to assess whether her complaints were due to amnesia, attention difficulties, or mood disturbance. She had notable difficulty with delayed recall of a word list with minor improvement with cues. There was an impairment of both semantic and phonemic fluency. Attention was variable, and she recorded mild depression and anxiety.
  ○ Bloodwork was obtained and her Vitamin B12, TSH, complete blood count (CBC), and liver function tests (LFTs) were within normal limits.
- Diagnosis: amnestic mild cognitive impairment

- o Rationale: Although the patient reports difficulties with executive function, on testing, she was noted to have more trouble with memory suggesting an amnestic profile. She has largely intact activities of daily living and therefore is diagnosed with mild cognitive impairment rather than dementia. Etiology is likely a combination of factors including mild vascular disease seen on MRI, poor sleep, anxiety, and depression, with a moderately high probability of early Alzheimer's pathology and a lower probability of limbic-predominant age-related TDP-43.
- Plan:
  - o We discussed lifestyle modifications including exercise, a healthy diet, maintaining social engagement, and making sure her blood pressure is under good control.[16,17]
  - o Sleep hygiene and improving sleep quality were recommended.
  - o We discussed observation versus starting an acetylcholinesterase inhibitor. The patient opted for the former option.
  - o We discussed testing to look specifically for amyloid using a PET-amyloid or lumbar puncture to confirm AD biomarkers, but the patient decided to take a "wait and see" approach as she has a good functional status.

CASE 2: ALZHEIMER'S DISEASE

- Chief complaint: "My husband has been telling me that I need to get my memory checked out."
- History: A 69-year-old woman with a history of hypertension and hyperlipidemia presenting for memory loss that has been progressive over the past few years. She does not think she misplaces items but her husband corrects her, stating that she does regularly and will accuse him of moving them. She will forget conversations and recent activities. She repeats herself. She denies word finding difficulties or getting lost but he notes she has gotten lost driving. She has difficulty multitasking and focusing on complex tasks. Family members note that she has had the same phone for a few years but sometimes she needs help when dialing calls. She denies anxiety or depression. They deny issues with her sleep.
- Activities of daily living: The husband reminds the patient to take her medications, and they developed a system to make sure she does not miss appointments. She stopped driving after a minor accident and is cooking less often than she used to after leaving the stove on a couple of times. The husband has taken over managing the finances.
- Family history: There is a family history of dementia on her father's side with onset in different family members ranging from age 66 to 80s.
- Physical examination: Cranial nerves were intact aside from decreased hearing on both sides. She had full strength and her sensation was equal to the examiner. No Parkinsonism was noted on examination.
- Cognitive testing: She scored a 17/30 on the MoCA. She missed three points for executive/visuospatial function, and one for fluency. She had 0/5 on recall and was only able to get two items with cues. She had difficulty with serial 7s and at one point forgot what she was subtracting. She missed one point for abstraction.
  - o Imaging testing: MRI was performed showing mild cerebrovascular disease with disproportionate hippocampal atrophy.
- Ancillary testing:
  - o apolipoprotein homozygous for E4 (APOE4) genetic testing: APOE4/E4.
- Diagnosis: AD in the setting of APOE4/E4 genotype with mild cerebrovascular disease.

○ Genetic testing was pursued given her young age and strong family history of AD starting in the late 60s. Patients with APOE4/E4 are three times more likely to develop late onset (after age 65) AD.

○ Rationale: Her clinical picture is largely amnestic in profile with some difficulty with executive function. The predominant amnestic profile coupled with the family history and positive APOE4/E4 genotype as well as hippocampal atrophy seen on MRI is consistent with AD. Mild vascular disease was also seen on MRI and is likely contributing to her symptoms. It is common that mixed pathologies cause dementia. Further diagnostic testing such as an amyloid PET or lumbar puncture (LP) was not performed given the high confidence in diagnosis.

• Plan:

○ She was started on donepezil and later, when her condition progressed to a moderate stage of dementia, memantine was added.

○ We discussed modifiable risk factors for dementia including exercise, a healthy diet, maintaining social engagement, and making sure her blood pressure is under good control.

○ She was referred to audiology for testing.

○ They were encouraged to start the process of obtaining a health proxy.

○ A referral was made to the Alzheimer's Association for resources for the patient and caregivers.

CASE 3: MILD COGNITIVE IMPAIRMENT: NON-AMNESTIC

• Chief complaint: "I'm not as sharp as I used to be."

• History: A 77-year-old woman with a history of hypertension, hyperlipidemia, atrial fibrillation with a pacemaker, obesity, and type 2 diabetes presenting with cognitive difficulties. She notes difficulty focusing and multitasking. Her friend says she is not repeating herself. She is under a lot of stress lately due to a family member trying to take over her mother's finances and she wanted to get elder services involved. The patient notes some anxiety, mostly associated with stress but denies depression. She occasionally mixes up the names of people and has missed taking some medications in the past but now has a reminder system in place. The patient has difficulty falling asleep and wakes up to use the restroom multiple times each night. She is not sure if she snores or is a fitful sleeper.

○ Family history: There is no family history of dementia, stroke, or seizures.

○ Activities of daily living: The patient pays her bills without mistakes, does her own cooking and cleaning, and has not mistakenly left the stove on. The patient is able to keep track of appointments. She denies any falls and walks a mile every day. She is able to successfully take public transportation to and from the grocery store.

• Physical examination: Cranial nerves, strength, and sensation are all within normal limits. She has a stooped posture but no shuffling when she walks or bradykinesia. Arm swing is symmetric.

• Cognitive testing: She performed 26/30 on the MoCA, missing two points for the visuospatial/executive function portion. It takes her several tries to register all five words then recalls three and the other two with semantic cues.

• Imaging testing: Recent head CT shows mild to moderate vascular disease, predominantly in the frontal lobes. There is mild global atrophy. There is no MRI as the patient has a pacemaker.

• Ancillary testing

○ Neuropsychological testing showed difficulty with frontal functions including difficulty with set-shifting, learning, abstraction, and problem-solving.

- o Bloodwork: Vitamin B12, TSH, and LFTs were within normal limits. Hemoglobin A1c was significantly elevated.
- Diagnosis: Mild cognitive impairment, non-amnestic type, and likely due to cerebrovascular disease.
  - o Rationale: History and diagnostic testing are most consistent with executive dysfunction rather than amnesia and the head CT along with a history of vascular risk factors support a diagnosis of cerebrovascular disease. Her activities of daily living are largely intact so she does not meet the criteria for dementia.
- Plan:
  - o We discussed lifestyle modifications including exercise, a healthy diet, maintaining social engagement, and making sure her blood pressure is under good control.
  - o The importance of glucose and blood pressure control to prevent further cerebrovascular damage was emphasized.
  - o Given the patient's high functional capacity, medications for the treatment of neurodegenerative dementia were not administered.

CASE 4: VASCULAR DEMENTIA

- Chief complaint: "I'm having memory issues and my thinking isn't as sharp as it used to be."
- History: A 74-year-old man with a history of atrial fibrillation, type 2 diabetes, hypertension, hyperlipidemia, and previous transient ischemic attack (TIA). His partner notes that he will ask the same questions just a couple of minutes later. He misplaces items. He was unable to learn how to use his new cellular phone. It takes him several minutes to put on his socks and get dressed in the morning and his partner notes that he knows what to do when dressing but is very slow. His TIA symptoms were difficulty speaking that improved after receiving a high dose of anti-platelet medication at the hospital. He snores and at times seems to cough and then awakens.
  - o Family history: There is a family history of heart disease and his father had two strokes.
  - o Activities of daily living: He stopped doing his finances a few years ago as he was prone to making errors. He stopped driving after a car accident and no longer goes shopping on his own.
- Physical examination: Cranial nerves are within normal testing parameters. Sensation is decreased in his feet. He has a right pronator drift.
- Cognitive testing: He scored 19/30 on the MoCA. He missed points, particularly in executive function and attention with impaired trail making, construction, verbal fluency, and serial 7s. He scored 1/5 on delayed recall but got two correct with semantic cues and two with multiple choice.
- Imaging testing: Brain MRI showed moderate-severe small vessel ischemic changes with two lacunar strokes.
- Diagnosis: Vascular dementia
  - o Rationale: Given the patient's numerous vascular disease comorbidities, executive dysfunction on history and examination, low score on MoCA, impaired activities of daily living, and brain MRI findings, he likely has vascular dementia.
- Plan
  - o Lifestyle modification including exercise, a healthy diet, maintaining social engagement.
  - o We discussed the importance of glucose and blood pressure control to prevent further cerebrovascular damage. The role of acetylcholinesterase inhibitors in

vascular dementia is mixed and after a discussion, we elected not to initiate them at this time.

- o Vascular dementia frequently co-occurs with AD pathologic changes and he will be monitored for progression.

CASE 5: FRONTOTEMPORAL DEMENTIA

- Chief complaint: "He's not the same person he used to be."
- History: A 62-year-old man with hypertension, hyperlipidemia, and major depressive disorder presenting with cognitive issues and behavioral changes. He endorses word-finding difficulties but otherwise denies any cognitive issues. His niece reports significant personality changes. He makes poor decisions including inviting prostitutes to the group facility where he lives and other sexually inappropriate behaviors that are out of character. The patient denies symptoms of depression, anxiety, mania, or auditory/visual hallucinations. He denies illicit substance use.
  - o Family history: There is no family history of similar disorders.
  - o Activities of daily living: There are no difficulties with basic activities of daily living but his niece has taken over the finances after poor financial decisions. He needs help cooking and shopping.
- Physical examination: He showed an inappropriate affect and lack of personal space. He paces the hallway waiting to be seen and gesticulates frequently during the interview. He laughs loudly at his own jokes. At times his speech is convoluted and his thought process is tangential. The examination is notable for normal cranial nerve, strength, and sensation testing. There is no evidence of parkinsonism. Frontal release signs are noted including brisk right palmomental and glabellar reflexes.
- Cognitive testing: 17/30 on the MoCA. He misses points on trails, cube drawing, clock drawing, repetition, serial sevens, date, year, and all 5 points on delayed recall.
- Imaging testing: A structural MRI was obtained. Imaging showed focal atrophy in the frontal lobes more than in the parietal lobes, and moderate temporal lobe atrophy. There were also mild white matter changes consistent with chronic small vessel ischemic changes. FDG-PET was obtained to better discern between frontotemporal dementia versus AD as a rare variant of AD can present with executive dysfunction. The scan showed decreased metabolism in the anterior cingulate cortex, frontal lobes, and anterior temporal lobes.
- Ancillary testing:
  - o Neuropsychological testing: formal neuropsychological testing revealed impaired working memory, cognitive flexibility, problem-solving, slow processing speed, learning, and verbal fluency. Thought processing was tangential and at times he was inappropriate or disinhibited.
  - o Bloodwork: Rapid plasma reagin (RPR) and human immunodeficiency virus (HIV) testing were negative. TSH and B12 levels were within normal levels.
- Diagnosis: Behavioral variant frontotemporal dementia
  - o Rationale: His inappropriate behavior, frontal release signs, executive dysfunction on examination, and brain MRI showing a preponderance of frontotemporal atrophy were consistent with a behavioral variant frontotemporal dementia. The pattern of decreased metabolism seen on the FDG-PET is more typical of frontotemporal dementia than typical or atypical variants of AD.
- Plan:

- o The patient was started on a selective serotonin reuptake inhibitor (citalopram) and referred for neuropsychiatry consultation where lamotrigine was added.
- o For safety precautions, residence in a skilled nursing facility was recommended.
- o The patient and family were referred to the Association for Frontotemporal Dementia

CASE 6: LOGOPENIC PRIMARY PROGRESSIVE APHASIA

- Chief complaint: Word finding difficulties and memory loss
- History: A 74-year-old woman from Puerto Rico, fluent in both Spanish and English, presents with progressive word-finding difficulties. The word-finding difficulty is worse in English than in Spanish. There may be stuttering and pauses in speech when searching for the right word. There are occasional erroneous word substitutions but the grammar is intact. The patient sometimes leaves the lights on and misplaces items around the house.
    - o Family history: Her mother developed memory loss in her 80s and was diagnosed with AD.
    - o Activities of daily living: She needs help managing finances and stopped driving due to getting lost multiple times.
- Physical examination: Cranial nerve examination is intact. She has mild bilateral apraxia shown as difficulty pantomiming gestures such as hammering a nail or screwing in a light bulb. There is no parkinsonism on examination.
- Cognitive testing: She scored an 18/30 on the MoCA. She demonstrated impaired visuospatial and executive function (poor cube copying and clock drawing) and decreased semantic fluency (reduced animal naming). Memory was largely intact (3 out of 5 recalled on the MoCA). She has obvious difficulty repeating phrases. In Spanish, she had impaired naming, scoring 4/15 on the short form of the Boston Naming test.
- Imaging testing: On brain MRI there was bilateral temporal lobe atrophy with enlarged Sylvian fissures and mild parietal lobe atrophy. An amyloid PET study showed symmetric amyloid deposition in the temporal and parietal lobes.
- Diagnosis: Logopenic primary progressive aphasia due to Alzheimer's pathology.
- Rationale: AD has multiple atypical variants including logopenic primary progressive aphasia and a visuospatial predominant form termed posterior cortical atrophy. Posterior cortical atrophy affects the parietal lobes and causes symptoms such as visuospatial dysfunction including difficulties understanding where items are in space or drawing as well as apraxia or difficulties with calculations. It can be caused by multiple pathologies but most often is due to Alzheimer's pathology. Logopenic primary progressive aphasia is one type of the three primary progressive aphasias and is also commonly due to Alzheimer's pathology. These patients exhibit impaired word finding and repeititon but have intact grammar and conceptual understanding of words. The other two forms of primary progressive aphasia are typically caused by frontotemporal dementia, with a non-fluent/agrammatic form that causes non-fluent aphasia and a semantic form that impairs knowledge of items (for instance, not only being unable to name a cactus but also not knowing where it grows, that it is known for having prickers, etc.). The primary progressive aphasias can be challenging to differentiate as all usually present with word-finding difficulties.[18]
- Plan:
    - o The patient was treated with donepezil and later memantine was added.

- o We discussed modifiable risk factors for dementia including exercise, a healthy diet, maintaining social engagement, and making sure her blood pressure is under good control.
- o It was recommended that a health proxy be established.
- o The patient and family were referred to the Alzheimer's Association for resources for the patient and her caregivers.

CASE 7: LEWY BODY DEMENTIA

- Chief complaint: Visual hallucinations and memory loss.
- History: An 80-year-old woman with a prior history of hyperlipidemia presents with memory loss, visual hallucinations, and attention difficulties. Her visual hallucinations started about 6 months ago whereby she sees little children or a man walking around her house. None of the hallucinations are frightening. The hallucinations are purely visual. In addition, she has difficulty remembering appointments and whether she took her medications. She has gotten lost walking outside of her building. She has fallen out of her bed at night while sleeping and gets lightheaded when she stands up. The patient is constipated and takes laxatives. She has had two falls and her walking pace is slow. Her handwriting is now smaller and more illegible. She is losing weight and does not eat much. When asked, she reports a decreased sense of smell.
  - o Family history: Her sister developed dementia of unclear type in her late 70s.
  - o Activities of daily living: The patient needs help with all of her instrumental activities of daily living and sometimes needs assistance when in the restroom.
- Physical examination: She has no resting tremor but has slowness of movement and mild rigidity. Gait is stooped but not shuffling. She has decreased arm swing on the left.
- Cognitive testing: The MoCA score is 10/30. There is difficulty understanding the visuospatial/executive function portions of the examination, only getting one point for clock contour. She has difficulty registering five words and gets one point on the recall subtest. Digit span forwards is intact but is abnormal backward, and the patient cannot do serial 7s. Naming is preserved but she only generates eight words on fluency testing. There is micrographia.
- Imaging testing: Brain MRI showed global atrophy without disproportionate hippocampal atrophy.
- Ancillary testing: Skin biopsy showed alpha-synuclein infiltration of the nerves.
- Diagnosis: Lewy body dementia.
  - o Rationale: The patient has a constellation of symptoms seen in Lewy body dementia including visual hallucinations, autonomic dysfunction, parkinsonism, likely rapid eye movement (REM) behavioral sleep disorder and decreased sense of smell. Approximately 80% of patients with Lewy body dementia develop visual hallucinations.[14,19] The diagnosis was confirmed on a skin biopsy showing alpha-synuclein infiltration of the nerve.
- Plan:
  - o The patient was started on an acetylcholinesterase inhibitor and had a significant improvement in hallucinations and cognitive impairment. She was not started on a carbidopa-levodopa medication which is commonly used in Parkinson's disease as she does not have a resting tremor. In addition, these medications are less effective in Lewy body dementia than in Parkinson's disease.
  - o A sleep study was obtained and REM behavior sleep disorder was found, which often co-occurs with Lewy body dementia. She was started on melatonin for treatment and referred to a sleep specialist.

- We discussed modifiable risk factors for dementia including exercise, a healthy diet, maintaining social engagement, and making sure her blood pressure is under good control.
- It was recommended that a health proxy be established
- The patient and family were referred to the Michael J Fox Foundation and Lewy Body Dementia Association for resources for the patient and caregivers.

SUMMARY

Diagnosis of subjective cognitive impairment, mild cognitive impairment, and dementia are all dependent on history including the patient's functional status, physical examination, imaging, and other ancillary testing. It is important to characterize the progression of symptoms as neurodegenerative causes of dementia are insidious. Many types of dementia can present with memory loss or word-finding difficulties so it is important to investigate whether the symptoms are associated with executive dysfunction or attention issues, mood dysregulation, true amnesia, language difficulties, or other medical problems. Presence of symptoms including visual hallucinations and parkinsonism should prompt a further diagnostic workup for Lewy body disease or Parkinson's dementia including a sleep study, possible dopamine transporter imaging, autonomic dysfunction testing, or skin biopsy. Behavioral changes raise concern for behavioral variant frontotemporal dementia. Brain MRI is useful in diagnosis to evaluate for atrophy, small vessel subcortical disease, bleeds, or other causes of altered cognition. Imaging including SPECT and FDG-PET is useful when evaluating for changes in regional brain function, particularly when differentiating frontotemporal dementia from other dementias. Biomarker studies may be useful to help confirm a diagnosis.

CLINICS CARE POINTS

- The progression of subjective cognitive impairment to mild cognitive impairment and dementia is based on objective cognitive testing and decline in the patient's ability to maintain instrumental activities of daily living.

- The most common cause of dementia is Alzheimer's disease followed by vascular disease, limbic-predominant age-related encephalopathy, Lewy body disease, frontotemporal dementia, and other causes. In elderly persons, mixed dementia pathologies are common.

- History, physical examination, imaging, and ancillary testing are all important when diagnosing dementia.

DISCLOSURE

Neither Dr S. Baratono nor Dr D. Press has real or potential conflicts of interest to disclose that pertain to the content of this article.

D.P. is supported by NIH grants R01MH117063, R01AG060987-0, R01AG060981 and is the site PI for clinical trials funded by Biogen and Janssen.

S.R.B is supported by NIH grants R56AG069086 and R01AG070077 as well as by the Sidney Baer Foundation 01028951 and Brightfocus foundation A20201288S.

REFERENCES

1. Rabinovitch GD. Late-onset Alzheimer disease. Continuum: Lifelong Learn Neurol 2019;25(1):14.

2. Galvin JE, Roe CM, Powlishta KK, et al. The AD8: a brief informant interview to detect dementia. Neurology 2005;65(4):559–64.
3. Jack CR, Bennett DA, Blennow K, et al. NIA-AA Research Framework: toward a biological definition of Alzheimer's disease. Alzheimer's Dement. 2018;14(4):535–62.
4. Pfeffer RI, Kurosaki TT, Harrah CH, et al. Measurement of functional activities in older adults in the community. J Gerontol 1982;37(3):323–9.
5. American Psychiatric Association, American Psychiatric Association DSM-5 Task Force. Diagnostic and Statistical manual of Mental disorders: DSM-5. 5th edition. American Psychiatric Association; 2013.
6. Mendez MF. Early-onset Alzheimer disease and its variants. CONTINUUM: Lifelong Learn Neurol 2019;25(1):34.
7. Nelson PT, Dickson DW, Trojanowski JQ, et al. Limbic-predominant age-related TDP-43 encephalopathy (LATE): consensus working group report. Brain 2019; 142(6):1503–27.
8. Seeley WW. Behavioral variant frontotemporal dementia. CONTINUUM: Lifelong Learn Neurol 2019;25(1):76.
9. Kumar N. Chapter 60 - neurologic aspects of cobalamin (B12) deficiency. In: Biller J, Ferro JM, editors. Handbook of clinical Neurology. Vol 120. Neurologic Aspects of systemic disease Part II. Elsevier; 2014. p. 915–26.
10. Elbadawy AM, Mansour AE, Abdelrassoul IA, et al. Relationship between thyroid dysfunction and dementia. Egypt J Intern Med 2020;32(1):9.
11. Geschwind MD. Rapidly progressive dementia. Continuum (Minneap Minn) 2016; 22(2 Dementia):510–37.
12. The Appropriate Use of neuroimaging in the diagnostic work-up of dementia. Ont Health Technol Assess Ser 2014;14(1):1–64.
13. Chen SJ, Tsai HH, Tsai LK, et al. Advances in cerebral amyloid angiopathy imaging. Ther Adv Neurol Disord 2019;12. 1756286419844113.
14. Armstrong MJ. Lewy body dementias. CONTINUUM: Lifelong Learn Neurol 2019; 25(1):128.
15. Kim JY, Illigens BM, McCormick MP, et al. Alpha-synuclein in skin nerve Fibers as a biomarker for alpha-Synucleinopathies. J Clin Neurol 2019;15(2):135–42.
16. Livingston G, Huntley J, Sommerlad A, et al. Dementia prevention, intervention, and care: 2020 report of the Lancet Commission. Lancet 2020;396(10248):413–46.
17. Middleton LE, Yaffe K. Targets for the prevention of dementia. J Alzheimers Dis 2010;20(3):915–24.
18. Botha H, Josephs KA. Primary progressive aphasias and apraxia of speech. CONTINUUM: Lifelong Learn Neurol 2019;25(1):101.
19. McKeith IG, Boeve BF, Dickson DW, et al. Diagnosis and management of dementia with Lewy bodies: fourth consensus report of the DLB Consortium. Neurology 2017;89(1):88–100.
20. Mayo AM. Use of the Functional Activities Questionnaire in Older Adults with Dementia. doi:10.3389/fnagi.2014.00255
21. Marshall GA, Zoller AS, Lorius N, et al. Functional Activities Questionnaire items that best discriminate and predict progression from clinically normal to mild cognitive impairment. Curr Alzheimer Res 2015;12(5):493–502.
22. Budson AE, Solomon PR. Chapter 2 - evaluating the patient with memory loss or dementia. In: Budson AE, Solomon PR, editors. Memory loss, Alzheimer's disease, and dementia. Second Edition. Elsevier; 2016. p. 5–38.
23.. Rascovsky K, Jodges JR, Knopman D, et al. Sensitivity of revised diagnostic criteria for the behavioral variant of frontotemporal dementia. Brain 2011;134: 2456–77.

Underlying Neuropathology and Basic Mechanisms

Neuropathology of the Common Forms of Dementia

Rupal I. Mehta, MD[a,b],*, Julie A. Schneider, MD, MS[a,b,c]

KEYWORDS

- Cardiovascular disease • Cerebrovascular disease • Dementia • Mixed dementia
- Neurodegenerative disease • Resilience • Resistance • Proteinopathy

KEY POINTS

- Dementia is a nonspecific term that corresponds to a group of heterogeneous, mostly age-related neurologic disorders that cause impaired cognition and deterioration of brain functions.
- This neurologic condition is a manifestation of various processes that primarily or secondarily affect the brain organ.
- Underlying neuropathologic substrates encompass various protein inclusions, vascular brain injuries, and cerebrovascular, traumatic, and metabolic brain changes.
- Protein inclusions and metabolic abnormalities accumulate in distinct stereotyped brain regions, whereas trauma and vascular-associated substrates may occur in patchy and/or irregular distribution(s).
- The burden and location(s) of brain lesions influence the type and degree of clinical symptoms, which establish the dementia syndrome.

INTRODUCTION

Dementia is an umbrella clinical term that refers to a range of debilitating neurologic conditions, and its incidence is increasing. Alzheimer disease (AD) dementia is the most common form of dementia.[1] However, a variety of neuropathological lesions are found in persons who succumb with dementia, including AD dementia.[2] Due to the chronic nature of dementing diseases and the range of potential causes and brain lesions, accurate diagnosis of dementia subtypes requires targeted postmortem brain dissection with comprehensive histologic evaluation and incorporation of ancillary testing. However, knowledge on complex causes for dementias also remains

a Rush Alzheimer's Disease Center, Rush University Medical Center, Chicago, IL 60612, USA; b Department of Pathology, Rush University Medical Center, 1750 West Harrison Street, Chicago, IL 60612, USA; c Department of Neurological Sciences, Rush University Medical Center, Chicago, IL 60612, USA
* Corresponding author. Department of Pathology, Rush University, Alzheimer's Disease Center, 1750 West Harrison Street, Chicago, IL 60612.
E-mail address: rupal_mehta@rush.edu

Clin Geriatr Med 39 (2023) 91–107
https://doi.org/10.1016/j.cger.2022.07.005
0749-0690/23/© 2022 Elsevier Inc. All rights reserved.
geriatric.theclinics.com

incomplete and, over the years, neurobiological and epidemiologic evidence have revised criteria used for neuropathologic diagnosis, scoring, and staging schemes. Similarly, neuropathological studies continue to inform on the significance of epidemiologic data and new forms of disease. Therefore, classification of this group of diseases is evolving.

A century of research has shown that various misfolded protein species accumulate in different brain regions and account for distinct proteinopathies that involve different susceptible cell types[1] Here, we explore the range of lesions that are documented within brains of persons who have died with a clinical diagnosis of dementia and summarize the causes, classification, topographies, and staging of these lesions. Although AD pathologic condition is the most common pathologic condition encountered overall, persons with AD type dementia (eg, amnestic dementia) may harbor multiple brain changes including various vascular pathologies and other non-AD neuropathologies, in addition to typical AD lesions. Other common forms of neurodegenerative diseases, such as those characterized by Lewy bodies and transactive response DNA-binding protein 43 kD (TDP-43) pathologic condition, as well as less common processes such as Creutzfeldt-Jacob disease and chronic traumatic encephalopathy (CTE) are described briefly. We also summarize nonproteinopathic diseases and mixed lesions that are linked to dementia syndromes. These other brain "hits" are recognized to lower the threshold for dementia in proteinopathic diseases.[3] Although summarizing current knowledge on dementia pathologies, this review also highlights knowledge gaps and emerging concepts pertaining to cognitive reserve.

PROTEINOPATHIC DISEASES

Proteinopathic diseases, also known as proteopathies or proteinopathies, are a heterogeneous group of protein misfolding disorders that manifest grossly as brain atrophy and histologically as accumulation of aberrant deposits within cortical or subcortical brain regions. These deposits selectively damage vulnerable neurons and/or glial cell populations in distinct brain regions, disturbing neural pathways and thereby altering brain structure and functions. Multiple mechanisms are involved, including neuronal and glial cell death pathways, organelle damage, and secondary physiologic disturbances including reactive astrogliosis and microgliosis.[4] Neuropathologic lesions accumulate chronically over time, thereby precipitating dementia syndromes. Primary diseases are listed in **Table 1** (upper panel) and are summarized below and in **Fig. 1**A, B, D.

Alzheimer Disease

Microscopically, AD neuropathologic change (AD-NC) is defined by the intraparenchymal accrual of 2 abnormal proteins, amyloid-beta (βA) in the form of extracellular plaques and irregularly phosphorylated forms of the microtubule-associated protein tau (MAPT), in the form of intraneuronal neurofibrillary tangles (NFTs).[5,6] On routine stains, these protein aggregates may seem as atypical eosinophilic inclusions within brain gray matter (for βA), or as irregular or flame-shaped intraneuronal inclusions (for NFTs; see **Fig. 1**A). These neuropathologic markers may be imperceptible on routine brain examination but are easily visualized on silver stains (eg, Bielschowsky, Gallyas, and Bodian) and/or via immunohistochemistry panels that incorporate primary antibodies targeted toward the aberrant βA or tau protein (eg, thioflavin S, AT8, Tau; see **Fig. 1**A). The abundance of these aggregates (especially tau protein) generally corresponds with the severity of cognitive impairment because they are related to variable degree of cortical brain atrophy, particularly in vulnerable medial-temporal lobe

Table 1
Summary of common diseases that lead to neurodegenerative lesions in persons with dementia

Disease	Etiologic Inclusion(s)	Primary Brain Regions(s) Involved
Proteinopathic Diseases Associated with Chronic Cell Loss		
AD-NC	β-Amyloid	Cerebral cortex
	Tau(3R and 4R)	Cerebral cortex
LB Disease	α-Synuclein	Brainstem and limbic region, including substantia nigra
LATE-NC	TDP-43	Hippocampus and temporal lobe
FTLD-Tau	Tau	Frontal and temporal lobes
FTLD-TDP	TDP-43	Frontal and temporal lobes
FTLD-Atypical	Ubiquitin, FUS[b]	Frontal and temporal lobes
PSP	Tau(4R)	Subcortical nuclei and brainstem, including substantia nigra
CBD	Tau(4R)	Cerebral cortex and subcortical nuclei, including substantia nigra
CJD	PrP	Hemispheric gray matter
HD	mHTT	Basal ganglia
PART	Tau	Hippocampus
CTE	Tau	Cerebral cortex
ARTAG	Tau	Cerebral cortex
CAA[a]	β-Amyloid	Cerebral cortex
Hippocampal sclerosis	TDP-43[c]	Hippocampus
Other Diseases Associated with Acute/Subacute or Chronic Cell Loss		
Cardiac and extracranial CVD	N/A	Global/multilobar/lobar, variable
Intracranial CVD (large vessel)	N/A	Global/multilobar/lobar, variable
Intracranial CVD (small vessel)	N/A	Subcortical gray or white matter, variable
Hippocampal sclerosis	N/A[c]	Hippocampus and white matter
Wernicke Korsakoff syndrome	N/A[d]	Mammillary body and white matter
Carbon monoxide poisoning	N/A[e]	Globus pallidus and white matter

[a] CAA may occur with or without AD-NC.
[b] FTLD-Atypical is characterized by FUS, ubiquitin, and neuronal intermediate filament inclusions, or basophilic inclusions.
[c] Hippocampal sclerosis may or may not be associated with TDP-43 and LATE-NC.
[d] The cause of Wernicke-Korsakoff syndrome is vitamin B1 (thiamine) deficiency.
[e] The cause of carbon monoxide poisoning is oxygen deficiency.

structures. Cerebral cortical and subcortical tissue loss leads to variable degree of symmetric sulcal widening, hippocampal atrophy, and lateral ventriculomegaly. AD-NC may also be characterized by the loss of neuromelanin-containing neurons in the locus ceruleus.

Extracellular plaques are formed by the accumulation and aggregation of βA with 40 ($^{1-40}$βA) or 42 ($^{1-42}$βA) amino acids. Aβ is a normal peptide product derived from cellular metabolism of the amyloid precursor protein (APP), which may be a neuroprotective molecule although its functions are yet unknown. APP undergoes sequential β-secretase and γ-secretase mediated enzymatic cleavage to produce amyloidogenic isoforms. Based on its accumulation pattern, βA-containing plaques are classified into

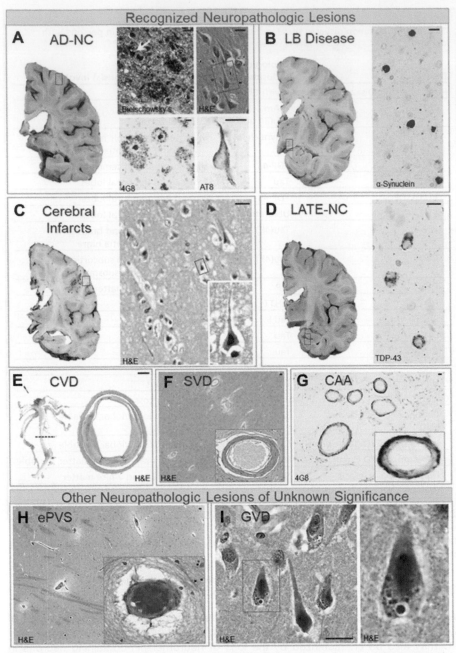

Fig. 1. Histologic features of common neurodegenerative disease lesions. (*A*) AD-NC is classically associated with frontoparietal atrophy (*left*). Etiologic lesions, shown at right (clockwise from *upper left*), include diffuse and neuritic plaques with neurofibrillary tangles (Bielschowsky's silver stain), neurofibrillary tangles (H&E stain), neurofibrillary tangle (phospho-Tau AT8 stain), and diffuse and neuritic plaques (4G8 amyloid stain). (*B*) LB disease is characterized by mild cortical atrophy with evidence of α-synuclein-positive LBs. (*C*) Macroscopic cerebral infarcts are characterized by cerebral edema with reperfusion-related

either diffuse plaques (DPs) or neuritic plaque (NP) varieties. NPs are composed of aggregated βA protein that may accumulate as dense cores and/or dystrophic neurites, which correspond to degenerated neuronal cell processes.[1–40] βA is enriched in NPs, whereas[1–42] βA is enriched in DPs. In addition to[1–40] βA, NPs also harbor variable numbers of astrocytic and microglial processes. βA NPs usually deposit in layers II–V of the neocortex but in advanced cases can also be noted in neocortical layers I and VI and in subcortical white matter.[7]

Tau protein, which is produced from MAPT gene, supports neuronal microtubule stability and is the primary constituent of NFTs. Alternate splicing of exon 10 generates tau species with either 3 or 4 conserved ~32 amino acid repeats (R), leading to either 3R or 4R tau on biochemical and immunohistochemical characterization. In AD, tau undergoes abnormal phosphorylation that promotes its aggregation into paired helical filaments.[8] These tau inclusions accumulate within neuronal cell soma as large rounded bodies and in neuronal dendrites and axons as neuropil threads.[8] The morphology of NFTs is variable because they acquire the shape of involved neurons. In cortical neurons, NFTs may be flame or triangular shaped (see **Fig. 1**A) but in subcortical or brainstem neurons, they are generally rounded and/or globose. Pre-NFTs exhibit diffuse, low-level tau label within the cytoplasm of intact neurons, whereas mature NFTs exhibit cytoplasmic filamentous tau aggregates that displace neuronal nuclei and extend into dendrites. Late-stage "ghost" NFTs seem entombed within nonviable, nucleus-devoid neurons.[8]

The successive accumulation of NFTs within the aging brain follows a stereotyped pattern that has been depicted in 6 stages.[7] Initially, NFTs are found only in the transentorhinal cortex (stage I and II). With disease progression, they gradually involve the entorhinal cortex and hippocampus (stage III and IV) and neocortical brain regions (stage V and VI; **Fig. 2**A). Similar to NFTs, βA accumulation also follows a stereotyped pattern of brain accumulation that is distinct from tau accumulation and has been described along 5 stages.[9] Initially, βA deposits within neocortex (stage I). With disease progression, they spread into allocortical brain regions such as entorhinal cortex, CA1, and subiculum region of hippocampus (stage II); subcortical nuclei including basal ganglia, thalamus, and hypothalamus (stage III); and, eventually into the medulla oblongata and midbrain colliculi (stage IV); and, finally, into pontine neurons and the cerebellar molecular layer (stage V; see **Fig. 2**A).[9] Although earlier staging schema required AD dementia for pathologic diagnosis of disease, revised guidelines for a diagnosis of AD-NC no longer require the presence of clinical symptoms. Current criteria for AD-NC require the presence of brain βA deposits. A diagnosis of AD is confirmed when there is at least intermediate or high AD-NC, which requires a Braak stage of 3 or more, and a Thal stage of 3. At this stage, most cases will have at least moderate NPs in the neocortex.

Lewy Body Diseases: Lewy Body Demenita and Parkinson Disease Dementia

Lewy body (LB) diseases are characterized by abnormal intracytoplasmic accumulation of alpha-synuclein protein positive LBs.[10] On routine stains, LBs seem as round,

---

petechial microhemorrhage (*left*) and acute neuronal necrosis (*right*). (*D*) LATE-NC is characterized by cortical atrophy with TDP-43-positive neuronal inclusions. Vascular changes and/or vascular brain injuries may also result from: (*E*) large vessel atherosclerosis, as depicted in the basilar artery; (*F*) SVD, such as arteriolosclerosis; and/or (*G*) CAA. Other neuropathological lesions of unknown significance include enlarged perivascular spaces (ePVS) and granulovacuolar degeneration (GVD), shown in (*H*) and (*I*), respectively. A–I: Boxed/marked area shown in enlarged and/or labeled section. Scale bars: A–D, F–I, 10 μm; E, 1 mm.

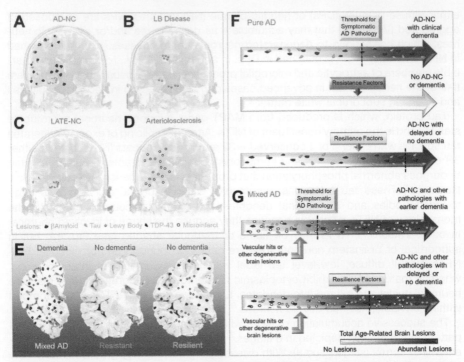

Fig. 2. Topographies and overlap of common proteinopathic and age-related disease substrates and effects on brain function. Topographic distribution of AD-NC (*A*), LB disease (*B*), LATE-NC (*C*), and arteriolosclerosis (*D*), which exhibit different susceptibilities. Mixed pathologic conditions (eg, βA plaques, Tau neurofibrillary tangles, Lewy bodies, TDP-43 inclusions, and/or cerebrovascular lesions) also occur (*E*). Persons who do not develop pathologic condition or do not progress to severe stage of pathologic condition are referred to as "resistant," whereas afflicted persons who do not exhibit dementia are referred to as "resilient." Various effects of AD-NC (*F*) and mixed pathologic conditions (*G*) are shown. Disease resistance refers to the absence of, or lower-than-expected disease burden, whereas resilience refers to the absence of, or delayed onset of cognitive impairment in the face of existing neuropathologies. (Agrawal and Schneider - Neuropathological Underpinnings of the Dementias. In Neuropsychology of Alzheimer's disease and other dementias, Second Edition.)

eosinophilic neuronal cytoplasmic inclusions that may be associated with peripheral halos and are highlighted by immunohistochemistry using antibodies directed to phosphorylated alpha-synuclein (see **Fig. 1**B).[10] When present in substantia nigra and accompanied by evidence of significant neuronal loss, these inclusions confirm a pathologic diagnosis of Parkinson disease (PD). With the involvement of cortical neurons, LBs may cause cognitive impairment and account for 2 recognized dementia syndromes, that is, Parkinson disease dementia (PDD) or LB Dementia (LBD). Although these disorders are similar, PDD is associated with cognitive changes typically occurring years after motor onset of PD, whereas LBD exhibits cognitive and motor (parkinsonism) impairment within a year of each other. Neuropathological data have demonstrated that accrual of LBs may progress along different anatomic pathways. Most frequently, LBs seem to ascend initially in pigmented brainstem nuclei (eg, vagus dorsomedial nucleus, locus ceruleus, and/or substantia nigra), and then along limbic areas (entorhinal cortex and anterior cingulate), and finally progress along neocortical brain tissue (**Fig. 2**B). Although presently unclear whether PD, PDD, and

LBD are truly distinct disorders or representative of a disease continuum,[11] pathologic condition is currently subclassified based on the regional LB distribution as brainstem, limbic or neocortical-predominant.[12] Postmortem evaluation shows that some brains feature LBs within the amygdala or olfactory bulb, but not brainstem, and these have been described as amygdala-predominant or olfactory types.[12] Spongiform change in entorhinal and other temporal cortical regions, and the presence of alpha-synuclein neurites within hippocampus CA2 sector and areas exhibiting LBs are supporting features of LBD. PDD and LBD may be associated with mild atrophy in affected brain regions. The observation of alpha-synuclein inclusions within glial cells characterizes multiple system atrophy.

Limbic-Predominant Age-Related TDP-43 Encephalopathy

Limbic-predominant age-related TDP-43 encephalopathy (LATE) is a recently characterized proteinopathy that afflicts older persons. LATE-neuropathological change (LATE-NC) is characterized by neuronal and glial TDP-43 inclusions in adults aged older than 80 years (see **Fig. 1**D).[13] LATE-NC includes neuronal loss and astrocytosis in the hippocampus with hallmark features of TDP-43 inclusions involving the limbic structures, olfactory bulb, basal ganglia, neocortex, and occasionally the brainstem. The TDP-43 inclusions initially present only in the amygdala (stage 1) but over time spread gradually to involve the hippocampus (stage 1 and 2) and midfrontal cortex (stage 3; **Fig. 2**C).[13] This neuropathology typically manifests with atrophy in mesial temporal lobe structures, including the hippocampus, and may occur concomitantly with hippocampal sclerosis (HS; described below). Indeed, most cases of HS in aging are associated with TDP-43 proteinopathy. The inferior frontal, and insular cortices, and other cortical regions may be less frequently involved.[13]

Hippocampal Sclerosis

HS is currently broadly defined as severe neuronal loss and gliosis of the hippocampus. In aging, it is most frequently neurodegenerative in origin. The vast majority of HS in aging is characterized by TDP-43 proteinopathy, hippocampal neuronal loss and/or gliosis[14] and thus is often part of LATE. HS is not specific to any other neurodegenerative disease pathologic condition but may be associated with several other classified disease processes, including various age-related neurodegenerative diseases (listed above), hypoxic/ischemic brain injury, and temporal lobe epilepsy.[15] In epilepsy, HS is often referred to as mesial temporal sclerosis. In neurodegenerative and hypoxic/ischemic diseases, HS is frequently characterized by severe neuronal loss and gliosis involving the hippocampus CA1 sector and the subiculum.[16]

Frontotemporal Lobar Degeneration

Frontotemporal lobar degeneration (FTLD) is characterized by cerebral cortical degeneration and is classified into 3 subtypes according to neuronal and glial protein aggregates.[17] FTLD-Tau exhibits hyperphosphorylated tau protein inclusions, whereas FTLD-TDP manifests TDP-43-positive protein inclusions, and FTLD-FUS exhibits fused in sarcoma protein inclusions.[17] FTLD-FUS includes atypical FTLD with only ubiquitin inclusions, neuronal intermediate filament inclusion disease, and basophilic inclusion body disease (BIBD), which are all characterized by FUS inclusions in addition to caudate nuclei atrophy.[15,18] Microscopic examination of brains exhibiting FTLD inclusions often show ballooned neurons, laminar spongiosis involving superficial cerebral cortical layers (ie, I–III), and prominent myelin loss in association with the above neuronal and/or glial cell inclusions.[17] FTLD also includes Pick disease, which is characterized by "Pick bodies" that seem as rounded, basophilic intraneuronal cytoplasmic bodies on routine stain and are composed of abnormally phosphorylated tau.[17] Unlike tau of AD-NC, the aberrant tau protein in Pick disease has been shown to form straight helical filaments and aggregates in frontal and temporal cerebral cortical neurons.[17] In addition to Pick bodies, cortical neurons in these regions also display ballooned neurons termed Pick cells.[17] As implied by its name, FTLD causes frontal and temporal lobe atrophy, which when severe is often described at knife-edge atrophy.

Progressive Supranuclear Palsy and Corticobasal Degeneration

Progressive supranuclear palsy (PSP) and corticobasal degeneration (CBD) typically present as atypical parkinsonian disorders but may also present with a dementia syndrome. PSP and CBD are characterized by NFTs involving the substantia nigra but unlike AD-NC, these diseases are characterized by 4R immunoreactive NFTs.[19] In PSP, 4R tau-positive tangles may additionally be found in subcortical regions such as the subthalamic and red nuclei, basal ganglia, and basis pontis.[19] In PSP, the 4R tau inclusions are also present in astrocytes and oligodendrocytes where they characterize so-called tufted astrocytes and coiled bodies, respectively. Tufted astrocytes display fine branching processes and may also be distributed within motor cortex. 4R tau-positive coiled bodies are also seen in subcortical white matter. In CBD, there is also 4R tau-positive tangles involving the substantia nigra but cortical pathologic condition is also prominent, especially in the perirolandic regions of the neocortex. In addition to neuronal tangles, CBD manifests with 4R tau-positive astrocytic plaques and neuritic threads in the cerebral cortex and subcortical basal ganglia, thalamus, and brainstem. Scattered achromatic or ballooned cerebral cortical neurons are typically present in the perirolandic cortices.[19]

Chronic Traumatic Encephalopathy

CTE describes the neuropathology associated with repetitive concussive and/or subconcussive head injuries, such as that which occurs in professional athletes including football and hockey players. This disease is characterized by neuronal NFTs present diffusely throughout the brain, including the hippocampus and brainstem, with accentuated perivascular distribution.[20] Perivascular and subpial glial tau accumulation may also be present. Grossly, CTE brains feature cerebral cortical and subcortical nuclear atrophy with enlargement of the lateral and third ventricles. CTE neuropathology has been shown to progress in 4 stages.[20] Initially, phosphorylated-tau NFTs deposits in perivascular NFT clusters, usually at neocortical sulcal depths (stage 1). Next, they accumulate in discrete clusters in perivascular and superficial cortical layers (stage 2). With subsequent progression, they aggregate multifocally in the medial temporal lobe, hypothalamus, thalamus, nucleus basalis, mammillary bodies, substantia nigra, raphe nuclei, and locus coeruleus (stage 3). Finally, with continued progression, NFTs distribute more widely throughout the brain and are associated with progressive myelin and myelinated axon loss (stage 4).

Huntington Disease

Huntington disease (HD) is a rare neurodegenerative disease that is caused by CAG (polyglutamine) expansion repeats in the huntingtin gene (ie, HTT) on chromosome 4.[21] Huntingtin protein misfolding causes intraneuronal aggregation of mHTT, primarily in striatal regions. Thus, this disease is characterized by striatal degeneration that is associated with secondary ventricular enlargement. HD is a familial dominantly inherited disease.[21] Neuropathological grading criteria used for this disorder is based on ventricle size and degree of striatal pathologic condition and atrophy.[22] Initially, only microscopic evidence of gliosis and neuronal loss is observed without gross evidence of striatal atrophy (grade 1). Disease progression features striatal atrophy with minimal changes observed early on in lateral ventricle size (grade 2) but there is increased striatal atrophy and ventriculomegaly with disease progression (grades 3 and 4).[22] Mild cerebral cortical neuronal loss may also be present and involve the frontal cerebral cortices.

Creutzfeldt Jakob Disease

Creutzfeldt Jakob disease (CJD) is a rare disease that is associated with various causes. The disease may be infectious, heritable, sporadic, or iatrogenic in nature.[23] CJD is characterized by intraneuronal prion protein (PrP) inclusions that induce severe and rapidly progressing neuronal loss and gliosis in various brain regions.[23] End-stage disease is usually characterized by severe cerebral cortical spongiform change and corresponding atrophy.[23]

Other Proteinopathies and Unclassified Tissue Changes

Other age-related neuropathologies feature neuronal and/or glial inclusions.[24] Argyrophilic grain disease,[25] aging-related tau astrogliopathy (ARTAG),[26] globular glial tau-opathy,[27] and primary age-related tauopathy[28] are also currently classified as separate neuropathologies. However, their epidemiologic significance and link to clinical dementia syndrome(s) is presently unclear. Moreover, the significance of other nonclassified (**Fig. 1**H) but well-recognized lesions such as granulovacuolar degeneration (**Fig. 1**I), which manifest in hippocampal pyramidal neurons of aged persons and commonly coexist with AD-NC, remain undefined.

AGE-RELATED VESSEL CHANGES AND VASCULAR DISEASES

Cerebrovascular pathologic conditions are common with aging and induce vascular and/or brain damage, both of which may contribute to structural brain pathologic condition.[29,30] Cardiac, extracranial and/or intracranial large vessel, and intracerebral small vessel diseases (SVD) may all contribute to dementia syndromes by compromising blood flow, causing subtle multifocal or diffuse neuronal dropout or more discrete, localized brain parenchymal injuries.[31,32] Thereby, these processes indirectly or directly lead to impairment of function in cognitive domains, although they may not directly induce deposition of intracerebral protein aggregates.[33] Although an array of disorders is recognized in this category, some older literature used nonspecific terminology to describe these lesions and no formal criteria exist for their grading or staging. Moreover, many cerebral SVD are only superficially classified, and their true incidences are unknown. A partial list of contributing disorders is summarized in the **Table 1** (lower panel), and described further below and in **Fig. 1**C, E–H.

Cardiac and Extracranial Cardiovascular Diseases

Cardiac diseases and extracranial cardiovascular disease (CVD; eg, structural or functional heart diseases such arrhythmic disorders, coronary artery, valvular, and/or hypertensive diseases, and extracranial carotid artery narrowing, occlusion, and/or emboli) are linked to ischemic phenomena with or without brain hemorrhage.[32] These diseases may lead to vascular brain injuries (VBI) including multifocal or diffuse ischemia with neuronal dropout and/or macroscopic or cystic infarcts (see **Fig. 1**C).[3] Mechanisms of cell depletion may include apoptosis and oncotic necrosis, among other mixed cell death pathways.[33] Although primary or secondary pulmonary or respiratory diseases such as chronic obstructive pulmonary disease, chronic obstructive sleep apnea, chronic bronchitis, and/or pneumonia, asthma, and/or pulmonary edema also compromise lung function and may contribute to hypoxia, their overall contribution to dementia syndromes remains controversial in the literature.

Intracranial Cerebral Large Vessel Diseases

Diseases involving the circle of Willis may also lead to VBI. Atherosclerosis (see **Fig. 1E**) and much less commonly large vessel vasculitis and other vasculopathies may cause hemispheric or focal ischemic stroke that leads to macroscopic cerebral infarcts, other macroscopic cystic infarcts, "strategic" infarcts, or contribute to microbleeds.[32] These diseases may also cause acute, subacute, or chronic neuronal dropout from hypoxic-ischemic damage. As with cardiac diseases and extracranial CVD, the mechanisms of cell depletion may include apoptotic, oncotic, and mixed cell death pathways.[37]

Intracerebral Small Vessel Diseases

Diseases involving cerebral small vessels also have potential to cause VBI, and recent studies emphasize the significance of cerebral SVD as a cause for neuronal loss, oligo-dendrocyte and myelinated fiber depletion, white matter rarefaction, microbleeds, small and microinfarcts, inflammation, and gliosis.[34,35] Arteriolosclerosis is the most common cause of cerebral SVD and causes partial or total fibrous replacement of intracerebral arteriolar smooth muscle cell layers (see **Fig. 1F**), with microbleeds and/or small and microscopic infarcts.[3,36] When widespread, this may lead to subcortical ischemic vascular disease, also known as multi-infarct dementia, Binswanger disease, or vascular dementia of Binswanger type (**Fig. 2D**).[36]

Cerebral amyloid angiopathy (CAA) is also common in older decedents and is characterized by βA deposition within basement membranes and/or smooth muscle cell layer of cerebral arteries and arterioles (see **Fig. 1G**).[37,38] This disease manifests with preferential deposition of [1-40] βA species and often leads to petechial microhemorrhages and less commonly lobar hemorrhage.[36] Severe forms of SVD results in vessel wall damage with vessel dilation, blood element extravasation, and occasionally vessel occlusion. Several community-based studies demonstrate an association of CAA with cognitive impairment.[39] Clinicopathological evaluations suggest significant associations between moderate and severe, multifocal CAA with ischemic pathologic conditions,[40] although a strong correlation is also noted between CAA and age. CAA commonly, but not always, accompanies AD pathologic condition and may also occur in the absence of significant AD.

Other Intracerebral Vessel Abnormalities

The prevalence of other uncharacterized and subtle vascular changes such as enlarged perivascular spaces [41,42] and blood–brain barrier disruption[43] in persons with dementia is increasingly recognized, although the significance of these changes is presently unclear (see **Fig. 1H**).

METABOLIC, TOXIC, AND OTHER DISEASES

Brain injury is also induced by a host of other diseases. Acute, subacute, and chronic metabolic disturbances are liable to contribute to dementia through various mechanisms. Additionally, metals and other environmental toxins may damage neurons through additional pathways.

Wernicke Encephalopathy and Wernicke Korsakoff syndrome

Wernicke diseases are precipitated by vitamin B1 (thiamine) deficiency.[44] Although recognized most commonly in association with chronic alcoholism, Wernicke

Korsakoff syndrome (WKS) is also observed in systemic diseases that result in nutrient deficiencies. In the acute phase, Wernicke encephalopathy (WE) is characterized by ophthalmoplegia, mental status changes, and ataxia, whereas the chronic phase of WKS includes confabulation and a dementia syndrome.[44] In WKS, bilateral mammillary body degeneration is observed on gross brain examination and is associated with hemorrhage and neuropil loss. With more extensive disease, WKS may be characterized by progressive involvement, including bilateral diencephalic degeneration.[44]

Carbon Monoxide Poisoning

Carbon monoxide poisoning is caused by inhalation of combustion fumes and binds to blood hemoglobin to form carboxyhemoglobin, which decreases blood oxygen carrying capacity and causes brain tissue hypoxia with preferential necrosis of the globus pallidus and subcortical white matter demyelination.[45,46]

Heavy Metals

Some evidence also suggests that dysregulation of metals such as aluminum, arsenic, and lead may precipitate dementia by causing oxidative stress with axonal and synaptic damage.[45]

AGE CONSIDERATIONS AND MIXED PATHOLOGIES

Among multiple potential causes described above, the most common causes of dementia are AD, CVD, and LB diseases (see **Figs. 1**A–C and **2**A, B, D), but proteinopathies may coexist with each other and with nonproteinopathic CVD/VBI lesions.[47,48] In fact, longitudinal cohort studies demonstrate that mixed pathologies represent the most common form of pathologic condition underlying age-related dementia including AD type dementia.[47,48] LB disease is reported to occur commonly with AD-NC, especially in persons aged younger than 60 years at death[49,50] but is also seen commonly in aging and with AD-NC.[51] As noted above, TDP-43 pathologic condition (see **Fig. 2**C) often coincides with HS and may also co-occur with LB disease.[52] Cohort studies have also shown that, in the oldest old, the incidence of AD-NC plateaus,[51,53] whereas other age-related pathologic conditions, specifically LATE-NC, become more common although the reasons for this are unclear. Despite the detailed diagnostic criteria summarized above for distinct neurodegenerative disease forms of dementia in aging, pure neurodegenerative diseases are relatively rare. Overlapping processes are thought to potentiate the common final pathway of neuronal loss and complex brain inflammation with gliosis that precipitate clinical dementia that is increasingly accepted as a multifactorial and pathologically heterogeneous disorder that occurs along a continuum with a range of phenotypes (**Fig. 2**E).[54] Overall, the location(s) and total burden of various neuropathological substrates determine the clinical dementia syndrome. Thus, the validity and utility of some classification and staging schemes for discrete neuropathologic forms of dementia in aging is presently unclear because mixed pathologic conditions are also recognized as a common cause for atypical clinical presentations. Interestingly, risk factors for dementia are also found to differ by age, with some CVD risk factors appearing to become protective in the oldest-old.[55]

LIMITATIONS OF CURRENT NOMENCLATURES, CLASSIFICATIONS, AND STAGING SCHEMES

Importantly, the above neuropathologies may also be present in persons who are cognitively intact.[56,57] In fact, in persons aged 90 years or older, 40% of individuals without dementia exhibit AD-NC or other neurodegenerative disease lesions.[55] In addition to recognition of mixed pathologies and age-related differences in epidemiology, it is increasingly accepted that coexisting proteinopathies and CVD/VBI potentiate dementia severity.[3,55,58] For example, LB, CAA, SVD, and VBI (see **Fig. 2**A–D) in many persons mitigate the burden of AD-NC required for the development of clinical AD-type dementia (**Fig. 2**F,G). Similarly, clinicopathological studies demonstrate that persons with overlapping AD-NC and LATE-NC tend to show more rapid cognitive decline compared with persons with pure disease[17,59] (see **Fig. 2**G). So, while data on the range of potential neurodegenerative disease substrates are advancing, epidemiologic data have also made clear that the presence of neurodegenerative pathologic conditions do not directly equate to dementia syndromes.[55]

During recent years, newer concepts have been introduced in attempt to explain the disconnects that are frequently observed between AD-NC score and degree of cognitive impairment, which presumably represent uncharacterized neuroprotective mechanisms. The term resistant is a heuristic that refers to persons whose brains remain "lesion-proof," or free of structural brain pathologic conditions throughout aging (see **Fig. 2**E, F).[60,61] In contrast, resilient is a term that refers to cognitive preservation, or the paradoxic ability to sustain cognitive function in the face of existing structural brain pathologic conditions[55] (see **Fig. 2**E–G). So-called nondemented individuals with AD neuropathology (NDAN), a.k.a. SuperAgers or asymptomatic AD [62] emphasize the significance of this group of elderly persons who are not prone to develop dementia and remain cognitively intact despite the presence of structural brain pathologic conditions (see **Fig. 2**E–G). Although both resistant and resilient persons have been said to exhibit cognitive reserve, evidence suggest that these are distinct phenomena that refer to unique scenarios, that is, resisting disease development versus compensating for existing disease(s).[61] The causes for these phenomena may include brain maintenance and neurorestorative factors that are presently unknown.[62] Emerging evidence indicate that lifestyle and behavioral factors, along with other metabolic, genetic, environmental, and/or physiologic variables, may influence AD-NC onset and progression, highlighting the importance of advising on nutrition, exercise, social, and cognitive activities, and control of vascular risk factors that may enhance cognitive functioning but are not accounted for in current classification and staging schemes.[21,55]

SUMMARY AND FUTURE DIRECTIONS

Dementia is very common in aging, and although AD pathologic condition (ie, AD-NC) is arguably the most common underlying pathologic condition, other pathologic causes of dementia in aging include Lewy bodies, TDP-43, vascular neuropathologies, and mixed pathologic conditions. Less common pathologic causes should also be recognized. It is important to note that each person has a different threshold for dementia onset. This threshold may be determined by various measures (e.g., the number of existing brain axons and synapses, neuroimmune state, stress level, and genetic and biological factors) and also often changes with age. New concepts and emerging data regarding cognitive reserve support the value of exploring nontraditional and/or nonstructural targets and risk factors for the purpose of preventing or delaying onset and progression of neurocognitive diseases in aging persons. Regarding current classification and nomenclatures, protein aggregates seem to be a final common denominator of many, but not all age-related dementia syndromes. Moreover, vascular mechanisms also play a fundamental role in many dementia syndromes. Indeed, it is notable that dementia syndromes also occur in the absence of protein aggregates, and what causes protein aggregates in the first place is incompletely known. With recognition of resistance and resilient factors and mixed pathologic conditions, the boundaries of distinct neuropathological diseases have become more uncertain. For these reasons, some experts have proposed a general neuropathological category of "brain dementia" in aging with specific lesions enumerated secondarily, whereas others suggest revision of current schema although evidence regarding precise revisions is lacking and the current schema continues to evolve.

What is currently known about dementia in aging is that: (1) Dementia represents a looming public health crisis.[1] (2) The brain undergoes various complex age-related structural, physiologic, and biochemical changes and is exposed to heterogeneous environmental stress conditions during the life span that may foster the development and progression, or resistance and resilience toward disease susceptibilities.[55] (3) In patients with dementia, a spectrum of neuropathologies contribute to neurodegeneration and may overlap. (4) Isolated and mixed pathologic conditions result in pruning and loss of neurons and glia and are associated with inflammation in various brain regions that collectively result in synapse and brain volume loss. (5) In persons symptomatic for dementia, the location(s) of neurodegenerative brain changes determine clinical symptomatologies. (6) Heterogeneity among clinical disease phenotypes indicates among other things, the existence of other nonclassified and or nonstructural determinants of disease.[55] Therefore, identification and investigation of potential nonclassified brain pathologic conditions, interactions of different brain pathologic conditions, and currently unrecognized resistant and resilient factors are required because they may not only elucidate hidden contributors to disease but may also uncover potential novel targets for disease prevention.

CLINICS CARE POINTS

- Alzheimer disease neuropathologic change is the most common dementia pathologic condition and manifests with diagnostic lesions of βA plaques and neurofibrillary tangles.

- Other common neuropathological forms of dementia include Lewy body disease, limbic-predominant age-related TDP-43 encephalopathy-neuropathological change, and vascular dementia.

- Additional pathologic conditions related to dementia include frontotemporal lobar degeneration, progressive supranuclear palsy, corticobasal degeneration, chronic traumatic encephalopathy, and Creutzfeldt Jakob disease, among others.

- Mixed and asymptomatic pathologic conditions are also commonly found in older persons.

- As modifiable risks, vascular diseases and lifestyle factors are important to address in the geriatric population but also show important age-related differences.

- Evidence suggests that traditional brain markers are not fully predictive of clinical disease because other physiologic factors affect the manifestation of dementia syndromes.

- Resistance factors prevent the appearance of neurodegenerative and other brain disease lesions, whereas resilience factors are hypothesized to mask cognitive dysfunction that would otherwise be predicted by the presence of a significant burden of neuropathologic lesions.

FUNDING

We thank the participants of the Rush Memory and Aging Project and Religious Orders Study and their families. This work is supported by P30AG072975 and R21AG079221.

DISCLOSURE

The authors declare no financial or nonfinancial conflicts of interest.

REFERENCES

1. Alzheimer's Association. 2022 Alzheimer's disease facts and figures. Alzheimers Dement 2022;18:700–89.
2. Brunnstrom H, Gustafson L, Passant U, et al. Prevalence of dementia subtypes: a 30-year retrospective survey of neuropathological reports. Arch Gerontol Geriatr 2008;49:146–9.
3. Kapasi A, DeCarli C, Schneider JA. Impact of multiple pathologies on the threshold for clinically overt dementia. Acta Neuropathol 2017;134:171–86.
4. Fiala JC, Feinberg M, Peters A, et al. Mitochondrial degeneration in dystrophic neurites of senile plaques may lead to extracellular deposition of fine filaments. Brain Struct Funct 2007;212:195–207.
5. Montine TJ, Phelps CH, Beach TG, et al. Alzheimer's Association. National institute on aging-alzheimer's association guidelines for the neuropathologic assessment of alzheimer's disease: a practical approach. Acta Neuropathol 2012;123:1–11.
6. Schneider JA, Arvanitakis Z, Leurgans SE, et al. The neuropathology of probable alzheimer disease and mild cognitive impairment. Ann Neurol 2009;66:200–8.
7. Braak H, Braak E. Neuropathological stageing of alzheimer-related changes. Acta Neuropathol 1991;82:239–59.
8. Moloney CM, Lowe VJ, Murray ME. Visualization of neurofibrillary tangle maturity in Alzheimer's disease: a clinicopathologic perspective for biomarker research. Alzheimers Dement 2021;17:1554–74.
9. Thal DR, Capetillo-Zarate E, Del Tredici K, et al. The development of amyloid beta protein deposits in the aged brain. Sci Aging Knowledge Environ 2006;2006:re1.
10. McKeith IG, Dickson DW, Lowe J, et al. Consortium on DLB. Diagnosis and management of dementia with lewy bodies: third report of the DLB consortium. Neurology 2005;65:1863–72.
11. Jellinger KA, Korczyn AD. Are dementia with lewy bodies and Parkinson's disease dementia the same disease? BMC Med 2018;16:34.
12. Attems J, Toledo JB, Walker, et al. Neuropathological consensus criteria for the evaluation of Lewy pathology in post-mortem brains: a multi-centre study. Acta Neuropathol 2021;141:159–72.
13. Nelson PT, Dickson DW, Trojanowski JQ, et al. Limbic-predominant age-related TDP-43 encephalopathy (LATE): consensus working group report. Brain 2019;142:1503–27.
14. Amador-Ortiz C, Lin WL, Ahmed Z, et al. D. W. TDP-43 immunoreactivity in hippocampal sclerosis and alzheimer's disease. Ann Neurol 2007;61:435–45.
15. Josephs KA, Whitwell JL, Weigand SD, et al. TDP-43 is a key player in the clinical features associated with alzheimer's disease. Acta Neuropathol 2014;127:811–24.
16. Ala TA, Beh GO, Frey WH 2nd. Pure hippocampal sclerosis: a rare cause of dementia mimicking alzheimer's disease. Neurology 2000;54:843–8.
17. Hernandez I, Fernandez MV, Tarraga L, et al. Frontotemporal lobar degeneration (FTLD): review and Update for clinical Neurologists. Curr Alzheimer Res 2018;15:511–30.
18. Josephs KA, Dickson DW. Hippocampal sclerosis in tau-negative frontotemporal lobar degeneration. Neurobiol Aging 2007;28:1718–22.

19. Mimuro M, Yoshida M. Chameleons and mimics: progressive supranuclear palsy and corticobasal degeneration. Neuropathology 2020;40:57–67.

20. McKee AC, Cairns NJ, Dickson DW, et al. The first NINDS/NIBIB consensus meeting to define neuropathological criteria for the diagnosis of chronic traumatic encephalopathy. Acta Neuropathol 2016;131:75–86.

21. Hong EP, MacDonald ME, Wheeler VC, et al. Huntington's disease Pathogenesis: two sequential Components. J Huntingtons Dis 2021;10:35–51.

22. Vonsattel JP, Myers RH, Stevens TJ, et al. Neuropathological classification of huntington's disease. J Neuropathol Exp Neurol 1985;44:559–77.

23. Watson N, Brandel JP, Green A, et al. The importance of ongoing international surveillance for Creutzfeldt-Jakob disease. Nat Rev Neurol 2021;17:362–79.

24. Brettschneider J, Libon DJ, Toledo JB, et al. Microglial activation and TDP-43 pathology correlate with executive dysfunction in amyotrophic lateral sclerosis. Acta Neuropathol 2012;123:395–407.

25. Braak H, Braak E. Argyrophilic grain disease: Frequency of occurrence in different age categories and neuropathological diagnostic criteria. J Neural Transm 1998;105:801–19.

26. Kovacs GG, Ferrer I, Grinberg LT, et al. Aging-related tau astrogliopathy (AR-TAG): harmonized evaluation strategy. Acta Neuropathol 2016;131:87–102.

27. Chung DC, Carlomagno Y, Cook CN, et al. Tau exhibits unique seeding properties in globular glial tauopathy. Acta Neuropathol Commun 2019;7:36.

28. Crary JF, Trojanowski JQ, Schneider JA, et al. Primary age-related tauopathy (PART): a common pathology associated with human aging. Acta Neuropathol 2014;128:755–66.

29. Arvanitakis Z, Capuano AW, Leurgans SE, et al. Relation of cerebral vessel disease to alzheimer's disease dementia and cognitive function in elderly people: a cross-sectional study. Lancet Neurol 2016;15:934–43.

30. Thal DR, Grinberg LT, Attems J. Vascular dementia: different forms of vessel disorders contribute to the development of dementia in the elderly brain. Exp Gerontol 2012;47:816–24.

31. Corrada MM, Sonnen JA, Kim RC, et al. Microinfarcts are common and strongly related to dementia in the oldest-old: the 90+ study. Alzheimers Dement 2016;12: 900–8.

32. Dolan H, Crain B, Troncoso J, et al. Atherosclerosis, dementia, and alzheimer disease in the baltimore longitudinal study of aging cohort. Ann Neurol 2010;68: 231–40.

33. Kahle KT, Simard JM, Staley KJ, et al. Molecular mechanisms of ischemic cerebral edema: role of electroneutral ion transport. Physiology 2009;24:257–65.

34. Poels MM, Ikram MA, van der Lugt A, et al. Cerebral microbleeds are associated with worse cognitive function: the rotterdam scan study. Neurology 2012;78: 326–33.

35. Hommet C, Mondon K, Constans T, et al. Review of cerebral microangiopathy and alzheimer's disease: relation between white matter hyperintensities and microbleeds. Dement Geriatr Cogn Disord 2011;32:367–78.

36. Smith EE, Schneider JA, Wardlaw JM, et al. Cerebral microinfarcts: the invisible lesions. Lancet Neurol 2012;11:272–82.

37. Auriel E, Greenberg SM. The pathophysiology and clinical presentation of cerebral amyloid angiopathy. Curr Atheroscler Rep 2012;14:343–50.

38. Grinberg LT, Thal DR. Vascular pathology in the aged human brain. Acta Neuropathol 2010;119:277–90.

39. Boyle PA, Yu L, Nag S, et al. Cerebral amyloid angiopathy and cognitive outcomes in community-based older persons. Neurology 2015;85:1930–6.
40. Akoudad S, Wolters FJ, Viswanathan A, et al. Association of cerebral microbleeds with cognitive decline and dementia. JAMA Neurol 2016;73:934–43.
41. Javierre-Petit C, Schneider JA, Kapasi A, et al. Neuropathologic and cognitive correlates of enlarged perivascular spaces in a community-based cohort of older adults. Stroke 2020;51:2825–33.
42. Mestre H, Kostrikov S, Mehta RI, et al. Perivascular spaces, glymphatic dysfunction, and small vessel disease. Clin Sci (Lond) 2017;131:2257–74.
43. Giwa MO, Williams J, Elderfield K, et al. Neuropathologic evidence of endothelial changes in cerebral small vessel disease. Neurology 2012;78:167–74.
44. Chandrakumar A, Bhardwaj A, t Jong GW. Review of thiamine deficiency disorders: Wernicke encephalopathy and Korsakoff psychosis. J Basic Clin Physiol Pharmacol 2018;30:153–62.
45. Killin LOJ, Starr JM, Shiue IJ, et al. Environmental risk factors for dementia: a systematic review. BMC Geriatr 2016;16:175.
46. Schofield P. Dementia associated with toxic causes and autoimmune disease. Int Psychogeriatr 2005;17:S129–47.
47. Boyle PA, Yang J, Yu L, et al. Varied effects of age-related neuropathologies on the trajectory of late life cognitive decline. Brain 2017;140:804–12.
48. Schneider JA, Arvanitakis Z, Bang W, et al. Mixed brain pathologies account for most dementia cases in community-dwelling older persons. Neurology 2007;69: 2197–204.
49. Beach TG, Malek-Ahmadi M. Alzheimer's disease neuropathological Comorbidities are common in the younger-old. J Alzheimers Dis 2021;79:389–400.
50. Beach TG, Adler CH, Lue L, et al. Unified staging system for lewy body disorders: correlation with nigrostriatal degeneration, cognitive impairment and motor dysfunction. Acta Neuropathol 2009;117:613–34.
51. James BD, Bennett DA, Boyle PA, et al. Dementia from alzheimer disease and mixed pathologies in the oldest old. JAMA 2012;307:1798–800.
52. Nag S, Yu L, Capuano AW, et al. Hippocampal sclerosis and TDP-43 pathology in aging and alzheimer disease. Ann Neurol 2015;77:942–52.
53. Robinson JL, Corrada MM, Kovacs GG, et al. Non-alzheimer's contributions to dementia and cognitive resilience in the 90+ study. Acta Neuropathol 2018; 136:377–88.
54. Jack CR, Therneau TM, Weigand SD, et al. Prevalence of biologically vs clinically defined alzheimer spectrum entities using the National institute on aging-alzheimer's association research Framework. JAMA Neurol 2019;76:1174–83.
55. Kawas CH, Legdeur N, Corrada MM. What have we learned from cognition in the oldest-old. Curr Opin Neurol 2021;34:258–65.
56. Hyman BT, Phelps CH, Beach TG, et al. National institute on aging-alzheimer's association guidelines for the neuropathologic assessment of alzheimer's disease. Alzheimers Dement 2012;8:1–13.
57. Serrano-Pozo A, Qian J, Muzikansky A, et al. Thal amyloid stages do not significantly impact the correlation between neuropathological change and cognition in the alzheimer disease continuum. J Neuropathol Exp Neurol 2016;75:516–26.
58. Korczyn AD. Mixed dementia–the most common cause of dementia. Ann New York Ann N Y Acad Sci 2002;977:129–34.
59. Nag S, Yu L, Wilson RS, et al. TDP-43 pathology and memory impairment in elders without pathologic diagnoses of AD or FTLD. Neurology 2017;88:653–60.

60. Bauckneht M, Chincarini A, Piva R, et al. Metabolic correlates of reserve and re-silience in MCI due to Alzheimer's Disease (AD). Alzheimers Res Ther 2018; 10:35.
61. Bocancea D, van Loenhoud AC, Groot C, et al. Measuring resilience and resis-tance in aging and alzheimer disease using residual methods: a systematic re-view and meta-analysis. Neurology 2021;97:474–88.
62. Kok FK, van Leerdam SL, de Lange ECM. Potential mechanisms underlying resis-tance to dementia in non-demented individuals with alzheimer's disease neuro-pathology. J Alzheimers Dis 2022;87:51–81.

Vascular and Nonvascular Mechanisms of Cognitive Impairment and Dementia

Betul Kara, MS[a], Marcia N. Gordon, PhD[a], Mahsa Gifani, MD[a],
Anne M. Dorrance, PhD[b], Scott E. Counts, PhD[a,c,d,*]

KEYWORDS

- Cognitive impairment • Dementia • Risk factor • Small vessel disease
- Neurovascular coupling • Proteinopathy • Oxidative stress • Neuroinflammation

KEY POINTS

- Cognitive impairment and dementia result from vascular and nonvascular processes that result in neurodegeneration and synaptic loss.
- Vascular mechanisms of cognitive impairment and dementia are related to small vessel diseases that manifest as dysregulated neurovascular coupling, blood–brain barrier function, and stroke.
- Nonvascular mechanisms of cognitive impairment and dementia are related to neurotoxic proteinopathies that disrupt multiple cellular homeostatic processes.
- Molecular mechanisms of vascular and nonvascular cognitive impairment and dementia include oxidative stress, mitochondrial dysfunction, and neuroinflammation.

INTRODUCTION

Cognitive impairment and dementia represent a significant departure from the trajectory of normal cognitive aging due to the aberrant accrual of pathogenic molecular and cellular pathway imbalances of vascular and nonvascular origins, which in turn lead to synaptic disconnection and neuronal loss in higher-order cognitive brain regions. This review combines data from foundational studies and recent breakthrough observations to summarize current thinking on several vascular, nonvascular, and common

[a] Department of Translational Neuroscience, Michigan State University, 400 Monroe Avenue Northwest, Grand Rapids, MI 49503, USA; [b] Department of Pharmacology and Toxicology, Michigan State University, 1355 Bogue Street, East Lansing, MI 48824, USA; [c] Department of Family Medicine, Michigan State University, 15 Michigan Street Northeast, Grand Rapids, MI 49503, USA; [d] Hauenstein Neurosciences Center, Mercy Health Saint Mary's Medical Center, 20 Jefferson Avenue Southeast, Grand Rapids, MI 49503, USA
* Corresponding author. Department of Translational Neuroscience, College of Human Medicine, Michigan State University, 400 Monroe Avenue Northwest, Grand Rapids, MI 49503.
E-mail address: countssc@msu.edu

Clin Geriatr Med 39 (2023) 109–122
https://doi.org/10.1016/j.cger.2022.07.006
0749-0690/23/© 2022 Elsevier Inc. All rights reserved.

mechanisms underlying the clinical presentation of Alzheimer disease (AD), vascular dementia (VaD), frontotemporal dementia (FTD), and dementia with Lewy bodies (DLB).

Genetic and Modifiable Risk Factors for Dementia

Dementia subtypes arise from multifactorial causes that likely involve interactions among biological aging, genetic factors, and environmental influences. Differential degrees of interaction among these factors may influence variations in age of onset, disease duration, and neuropathological patterns underlying dementia subtypes.[1]

AD is a polygenic disorder with multiple genetic components affecting the likelihood of disease onset and people who have a first-degree relative with AD are more likely to succumb to the disease.[2] Familial forms of AD (<5% cases) are inherited in an autosomal dominant manner through point-mutations and deletion-mutations in *PSEN1*, *PSEN2*, and *APP* genes and result in early-onset AD (EOAD), typically presenting during the fourth to sixth decade of life.[2] The mutated EOAD gene products are all dysfunctional in the sequential cleavage of the amyloid precursor protein (APP) to produce amyloid-β (Aβ) peptides, which aggregate to form the nidus of amyloid plaque pathology (see later discussion).[1] Late-onset AD (LOAD, age > 65), however, is significantly associated with several genetic risk factors, with the inheritance of the *APOE* ε4 allele increasing disease likelihood and lowering age of onset by dysregulating lipid transport, altering blood–brain barrier (BBB) permeability, and promoting vascular amyloid deposition.[3] Other factors that confer risk for LOAD include single nucleotide polymorphisms in *CLU, PICALM, CR1, BIN1, ABCA7, CD2AP, CD33, EPHA1*, and the *MS4A* cluster.[4,5] Many of these genes encode components of innate immunity pathways in the brain.

By contrast, ~40% of FTD patients have a positive family history with ~10% demonstrating an autosomal dominant inheritance pattern.[6] To date, more than 10 genes have been linked to FTD, with *MAPT, PGRN*, and *C9orf72* accounting for ~60% of familial FTD.[7] Less common mutations associated with familial FTD occur in the *VCP, CHMP2B, TARDBP, FUS, SQSTM1, CHCHD10, TBK1, OPTN, CCNF*, and *TIA1* genes, which cumulatively account for less than 5% of all FTD cases.[8] Regarding potential mechanisms of disease related to these mutations, it is notable that *MAPT* encodes the tau protein involved in tauopathies, whereas *PGRN* (encoding progranulin) and *TARDBP* (encoding TAR DNA binding protein 43 [TDP-43]) result in TDP-43 pathologic conditions in FTD (see later discussion).

The genetic basis of DLB is elusive yet there is potential genetic overlap between DLB, FTD, and AD. For example, *PSEN1* mutations have also been detected in DLB and FTD patients.[9,10] Similarly, mutations in *MAPT, PGRN*, and *C9orf72* have been found in patients diagnosed with DLB and AD.[11,12] Moreover, *APOE* ε4 inheritance also influences risk for DLB and FTD,[13,14] and mutations in the *SCNA* and *GBA* genes associated with Parkinson disease (PD) are associated with DLB.[15] However, the extent to which these genes are linked independently to multiple dementing disorders or represent mixed dementia causes remains unclear.

Finally, mutations in the *NOTCH3* gene result in cerebral autosomal dominant arteriopathy with subcortical infarct and leukoencephalopathy (CADASIL). The *NOTCH3*-encoded protein directs cell fate, and CADASIL-associated mutations result in smooth muscle cell degeneration as well as pericyte and endothelial cell dysfunction, resulting in impaired permeability and perfusion and, ultimately, multiple subcortical strokes and VaD (~30% of patients aged younger than 60 years).[16]

Nongenetic factors associated with dementia include age, sex, and modifiable comorbidities arising from environmental and lifestyle factors. For instance, the Lancet

Commission, an international panel of dementia epidemiology experts, identified 12 modifiable risk factors across the life span that, irrespective of diet, collectively increase the risk for dementia by ~40%: less education (early life); hypertension, obesity, hearing loss, traumatic brain injury, and alcohol abuse (midlife, ages ~45–66 years); and physical inactivity, diabetes, social inactivity, depression, smoking, and air pollution (late life).[17]

Vascular Mechanisms of Dementia

Dementia was considered a vascular disease for decades before the identification of AD-related plaque and tangle pathologic conditions,[18] after which the consideration of vascular causes of dementia lost attention. Two key findings brought vascular contributions to cognitive impairment and dementia back to the forefront: (1) the observation that dementia occurring purely because of vascular injury or dysfunction (ie, VaD) accounts for 10%–20% of dementia cases, and (2) the discovery that all major forms of dementia have a vascular component that exacerbates the disease.[19] The vascular component of dementia frequently takes the form of cerebral small vessel disease (SVD),[20] which can manifest as poststroke dementia, subcortical vascular encephalopathy, strategic and multi-infarct dementia, and/or mixed dementia[21] through mechanisms involving excitotoxicity, reactive oxygen species generation, BBB breakdown, neuroinflammation, and cell death.[22]

Hypertension is a leading cause of cerebral SVD and a modifiable risk factor for the development of dementia.[23] Regulating blood pressure to less than 140 mm Hg reduces dementia risk[24] and lowering blood pressure less than 120 mm Hg reduces the white matter hyperintensities and brain atrophy associated with dementia.[25] The deleterious effects of hypertension on brain perfusion are a clear mechanistic link to dementia risk. The brain has a limited capacity to store energy, so when localized neural activity increases, blood flow to that region must follow suit. This functional hyperemic response provides the oxygen and glucose needed for neuronal function while also removing the metabolites produced by neuronal activity. This process, known as neurovascular coupling, is impaired in patients with hypertension.[26]

Capillaries are the smallest segments of the cerebral vascular bed, yet dysfunction in their role in gas and nutrient exchange is likely to affect cognitive function. Capillary endothelial cells play a central role in activating the mechanisms that drive neurovascular coupling. Neuronal activity increases extracellular potassium, which causes a retrograde hyperpolarization of the capillary cells up to the arterioles, where it produces dilation, thereby increasing blood flow to the capillary bed.[27] Recent studies have shown that conducted vasodilation and neurovascular coupling are impaired in blood pressure high (BPH)/2 genetically hypertensive mice and can be corrected by normalizing blood pressure with a calcium channel blocker.[28]

Parenchymal arterioles (PAs) branching from the pial vessels are also important determinants of cognitive function. PAs are not connected by collateral branches, and the occlusion of a single PA is sufficient to produce cognitive impairment.[29] Thus, PAs are often described as a weak link in an otherwise resilient vascular system.[30] PAs account for 30% to 40% of cerebrovascular resistance,[31] so small reductions in PA dilator capacity can significantly impair the perfusion of the white matter, which receives most of its blood supply through these arterioles.[30]

We have linked impaired endothelium-dependent dilation to the transient receptor potential vanilloid 4 (TRPV4) ion channel,[32] which transports calcium into the endothelial cells to activate endothelium-dependent hyperpolarization and regulate blood flow.[33] We have shown that inhibiting soluble epoxide hydrolase (sEH), which reduces the activity of epoxyeicosatrienoic acid TRPV4 ligands, improves cognitive function in a model of hypertensive chronic cerebral hypoperfusion.[34] Importantly, sEH expression is increased in patients with VaD and sEH inhibition improves cognitive function in models of AD.[35]

Finally, reduced vascular capacity for the clearance of waste from the brain to cervical lymph nodes may represent another mechanism conferring dementia risk. In addition to impairments in neurovascular coupling driven by SVD such as hypertension, impairments in the glymphatic system, which facilitates perivascular drainage of waste products from the brain by arterial pulsation,[36] and intramural periarterial drainage, which clears waste—including soluble proteins such as Aβ—along the basement membranes of smooth muscle cells,[37] have gained attention. In this regard, glymphatic clearance is also perturbed in hypertensive models.[38] Thus, there are multiple mechanisms by which cerebral SVD and associated vascular lesions impact the development of dementia.

Nonvascular Mechanisms of Dementia—Proteinopathies

A notable commonality among nonvascular dementias is the spectrum of proteinopathies—or accrual of aggregated protein deposits—that define these disorders. Despite variability in the specific protein involved and differential spatiotemporal patterns of deposition, proteinopathies share pathologic signatures including beta-sheet fibrillar aggregates, "prion-like" spread in the brain, activation of immune responses, and evidence for disease-related deficits in clearance.[39] Overlapping proteinopathies are also common despite a clinical presentation suggesting a singular disease (eg, many patients diagnosed antemortem with AD display mixed pathologic conditions on postmortem evaluation).[40] The 4 most relevant proteinopathies are tauopathy, amyloid pathology, synucleinopathy, and TDP-43 pathology.

Tauopathies including AD and FTD subtypes such as behavioral variant FTD (bvFTD), corticobasal degeneration (CBD), and progressive supranuclear palsy are characterized by intracellular neurofibrillary tangle (NFT) accumulation comprising highly phosphorylated moieties of the protein tau (the product of *MAPT*). Tau is a microtubule-binding protein predominantly located in the axon. Besides its function in microtubule stabilization in the axon, monomeric tau is involved in multiple cellular pathways including cell signaling.[41] Tauopathy is variably accompanied by other proteinopathies including amyloid pathology in AD, synucleinopathy in DLB and AD, and TDP-43pathology in FTD (see later discussion). Although the cascade of events leading from monomeric tau to NFTs is not fully known, oligomeric tau intermediates confer neurotoxicity through a diverse array of mechanisms including the impairment of synaptic function and long-term potentiation (LTP) resulting in learning and memory deficits,[42] autophagic-lysosomal pathways resulting in the accumulation of damaged proteins and mitochondrial dysfunction,[43] axonal trafficking,[41] and genomic stability.[44]

Amyloid pathology in the form of plaques and amyloid angiopathy in AD and DLB results from the aggregation of Aβ peptides. Similar to tau, Aβ toxicity seems to be due to soluble, diffusible oligomeric (oAβ) intermediates. oAβ also impairs LTP, possibly through overactivation of NMDA receptors.[45] oAβ-mediated LTP impairment has also been linked to Ca^{2+} dyshomeostasis, mitochondrial dysfunction, and oxidative stress.[46] oAβ also mediates neuronal excitotoxicity by increasing presynaptic glutamate release and disrupting postsynaptic glutamate receptor function.[47] Intriguingly, oAβ was found to promote hyperphosphorylation of tau by activating tau kinases, which leads to the formation of NFTs.[46] Finally, oAβ also impairs insulin signaling, which plays a role in Aβ clearance from the brain.[48]

Synucleinopathy arises from the aggregation of the presynaptic protein α-synuclein (α-syn, the protein product of *SCNA*).[49] Fibrillar aggregates of α-syn are the major constituents of Lewy bodies, the pathologic hallmark of Lewy body diseases including dementing subtypes such as DLB and PD with dementia.[50] Functionally, α-syn seems to regulate presynaptic vesicle transport by binding SNARE complexes.[51] Pre-Lewy body oligomeric forms of α-syn (o-α-syn) cause cellular toxicity via mechanisms including damage to mitochondrial respiration and ATP production[52] with resulting increases in oxidative stress.[53] O-α-syn has also been linked to disruptions of the autophagic-lysosomal pathway,[54] which in turn likely results in the further accumulation of pathologic aggregates of α-syn. Along with synucleinopathy, amyloid pathology is another feature of DLB[50]; however, the extent to which these 2 proteinopathies independently or synergistically promote disease progression remains undefined.

Another proteinopathy consists of the nuclear TDP-43 (the protein product of *TARDBP*). TDP-43 aggregates are associated with FTD subtypes including bvFTD and CBD (both with concomitant tauopathy) and amyotrophic lateral sclerosis.[55] TDP-43 pathology is also commonly seen in AD[56] and the recently recognized dementia subtype, limbic-predominant age-related TPD-43 encephalopathy (LATE).[57] These disorders display cytoplasmic phosphorylated and ubiquitinated TDP-43 inclusions that strongly correlate with neurodegeneration.[55,57] Physiologically, TDP-43 orchestrates RNA splicing, transport, and translation,[55] so clinically distinct neurologic diseases associated with cytoplasmic TDP-43 inclusions may be related to impaired chromatin remodeling, RNA metabolism, and impaired mitochondrial and stress–response pathways such as the endoplasmic reticulum unfolded protein response.[58]

Common Mechanisms of Dementia—Oxidative Stress and Mitochondrial Dysfunction

Oxidative stress is a common theme among proteinopathies (eg, oxidative/nitrative damage to tau, Aβ, α-syn, and TDP-43 may promote their aggregation)[59,60] and/or vascular damage (as part of the ischemic cascade).[18] The brain is at particular risk for oxidative damage because it uses 20% of the body's oxygen supply and yet is relatively depleted of antioxidant defenses (eg, brain tissue production of catalase is ~10%–20% of that in liver and heart).[61] Notably, even subjects who come to autopsy with mild cognitive impairment (MCI), a putative prodromal stage of AD and related dementias, display differential cellular levels of macromolecular oxidative damage, decreased antioxidant defenses, and mitochondrial dysfunction, underscoring the potentially prominent pathogenic role for dysregulated redox balance and cellular respiration during disease progression.[59,62,63]

Oxidative stress associated with MCI and AD includes: (1) protein carbonylation produced by amino acid oxidation or advanced glycation end product formation, (2) protein nitrosylation from superoxide radicals reacting with nitric oxide, (3) nuclear and mitochondrial DNA as well as RNA oxidation from hydroxyl radical damage, and (4) lipid peroxidation such as F_2-isoprostanes and F_4-isoprostanes and hydroxynonenal (HNE) aldehyde protein adducts in key cognitive regions such as hippocampus and cortex.[59,63–65] Oxidative stress markers have also been noted in plaques and NFTs.[66]

Increased lipid peroxidation and HNE were also noted in FTD.[67] Stem cell-derived neurons bearing tau mutations from patients with FTD and parkinsonism linked to chromosome 17 displayed mitochondrial perturbations including reduced respiration and lower ATP production, which in turn were associated with higher levels of superoxide production and lipid peroxidation compared with control neurons.[68] Oxidative stress and mitochondrial dysfunction are also associated with DLB as studies using frozen cortex from patients revealed dysregulation of mitochondrial subunit expression and reduced activity of complexes I, II, III, and IV of the respiratory chain.[69] Oxidative damage in DLB has also been noted in the widespread distribution of neurons and glia bearing markers for protein nitration[70] and higher cortical levels of oxidized cholesterol compared with controls,[71] as well as oxidation and nitration of reflect Greek alpha and Lewy bodies.[66]

The mechanisms underlying increased oxidative stress remain unclear. Normal cellular metabolism produces low concentrations of reactive oxygen species and reactive aldehydes (eg, HNE), which play important roles as signaling molecules to regulate cell differentiation, cell signaling, cell survival, and immune responses.[72] However, cell damage could be perpetuated by feed-forward cycles whereby increased oxidative stress leads to damaged mitochondrial DNA and respiratory chain subunits resulting in impaired mitochondrial function and increased levels of free radicals.[73] Notably, MCI is also characterized by impaired mitochondrial biogenesis, increased fission and mitophagy, and aberrant mitochondrial unfolded protein responses.[73,74] Vascular contributions to cognitive impairment and dementia also involve mitochondrial stress and dysfunction from focal hypoxia, which may trigger this vicious cycle via pro-oxidant enzymes such as NADPH oxidase 1.[75] In addition, the relatively insufficient antioxidant defense system of the brain is further compromised during disease pathogenesis. For instance, others and we have shown that the expression levels of antioxidant enzymes such as glutathione peroxidase and superoxide dismutase are significantly reduced in plasma and vulnerable brain regions in MCI/AD.[62,76,77] Furthermore, in vivo imaging studies have shown that reduced brain glutathione levels correlate with poorer cognitive performance in MCI and AD subjects.[78]

Finally, cellular loss of ATP from dysfunctional mitochondria leads to dysregulated ion gradients and membrane depolarization resulting in impaired action potentials and Ca^{2+} dyshomeostasis.[79] Hence, the cumulative toll of oxidized DNA/RNA, oxidative/nitrative protein damage, mitochondrial dysfunction, and impaired ATP production is the significant perturbation of synaptic activity necessary for maintaining cognitive function.[18,73,79] Finally, oxidative stress is also associated with increased neuroinflammation by driving glial expression of proinflammatory cytokines and transcription factors, as described below.

Common Mechanisms of Dementia—Neuroinflammation

Abnormal, silver-stained glial cells were among the pathologic conditions noted in the first, seminal reports from Dr Alzheimer. Modern immunohistochemical methods subsequently detailed increased immune system-related proteins produced by reactive microglia and astrocytes in AD, including complement proteins, major histocompatibility complex I and II proteins, integrins such as CD11b and CD18, and a myriad of proinflammatory cytokines such as interleukins IL-1β and IL-6 and the tumor necrosis factor, TNFα.[80,81] Binding of these integrins and cytokines to their cognate receptors initiates second messenger pathways (eg, MAP and JUN kinases, nuclear factor-kappa B activator protein 1 transcription factors) to induce immune amplification via the production of additional cytokines, chemokines, reactive oxygen and nitrogen species, prostaglandins, proteolytic enzymes, and a variety of other factors, which can even result in apoptosis or necrosis.[82–84]

These glial changes were initially thought to represent cellular responses to amyloid plaques and NFTs and/or degenerating neurons. However, a paradigm shift from the concept of "reactive gliosis" occurred when multiple genome-wide association studies (GWAS) involving tens to hundreds of thousands of subjects identified 30 to 50 single nucleotide polymorphisms linked to AD risk, with a large proportion associated with immune function.[85] More recently, a landmark GWAS study involving 111,326 AD cases and 677,663 controls identified 75 total polymorphisms associated with disease risk, among which 33 were novel and primarily associated with microglial function and TNFα pathways.[86] Considered together, these data suggest that glial functions could contribute to causing disease pathogenesis, rather than merely responding to it. Neuroinflammation is hypothesized to be a major component of FTD[87] and LBD,[88] as well as in VaD where inflammatory responses are associated with hypertension, BBB damage, and stroke.[18] Here, we will focus on neuroinflammation in AD because this has been extensively researched and likely involves mechanisms common among dementia subtypes.

With respect to alterations in glial cells in AD and related dementias, transcriptomic signatures identified subtypes of microglia and astrocytes associated with disease and injury.[89] In microglia, these cells have been termed "disease-associated microglia" (DAM)[90] and "microglia associated with neurodegeneration" (MGnD).[91] DAM/MgNDs display reductions in homeostatic genes and increases in genes associated with innate immune activation and genetic risk factors for AD. Two genetic risk factors for AD, APOE and triggering receptor expressed on myeloid cells 2 (TREM2), are required for the conversion from the homeostatic to the DAM/MGnD phenotype.[91] The activated microglia secrete factors such as C1q, interleukin IL-1α, and TNFα that induce astrocyte activation to the neurotoxic, reactive A1 phenotype.[92] Interestingly, the secondary structure of Aβ is sufficient to interact with microglial receptors such as TREM2 and toll-like receptors, directly stimulating innate immunity secretory pathways and phagocytosis.[93] Because amyloid pathology in AD accumulates late in the life span, there could be no selection pressure on microglia to evolve specific mechanisms for Aβ removal. This likely represents another impaired clearance mechanism for amyloid and may be relevant for other proteinopathies.

Complement activation is another critical arm of innate immunity. Initially, complement C1q binds to a target antigen and initiates a cascade of protease activation. Cleavage products C3b and C4b "opsonize" structures, tagging them for removal by phagocytes such as microglia, while other cleavage products, C3a and C5a, elicit cytokine secretion, B cell stimulation, smooth muscle contraction, and capillary leakage.[94] The Aβ peptide is capable of binding C1q and activating the complement cascade.[95] oAβ causes some synapses to become decorated with C1q, which triggers opsonization by C3 and synaptic stripping and may play a key role in the presentation of dementia.[96,97] Genetic or pharmacologic interruption of C1q, C3, or C5 signaling prevented synapse loss, cognitive impairment and, in some situations, amyloid accumulation in mouse models.[96–98]

Complement activation may also play a role in VaD and is related to both chronic hypoperfusion[99] and amyloid angiopathy.[100] Notably, cross talk between complement and coagulation pathways results in prothrombic roles for both C3a and C5a.[94] Human cerebrovascular smooth muscle cells secrete complement proteins leading to lytic injury, loss of vessel integrity, and potentially even exacerbating amyloid angiopathy and cognitive function.[101] In addition, genetic deletion or pharmacologic antagonism of C3a receptors protected against cerebral ischemia caused by bilateral common carotid stenosis in a mouse model of VaD.[102]

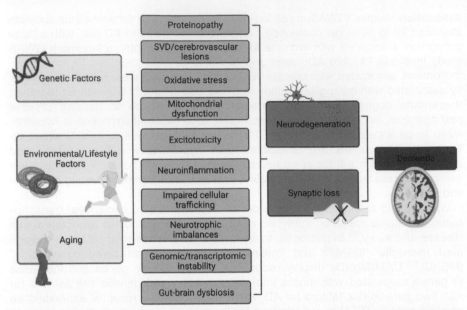

Fig. 1. Pathogenic mechanisms of cognitive impairment and dementia. Aging, familial gene mutations, genetic risk factors, and potentially modifiable risk factors related to lifestyle or environmental exposures interact to predispose individuals to cognitive impairment or dementia to different degrees by influencing the efficacy of multiple, often interdependent cellular and molecular pathways. The extent to which these pathways are shifted from homeostatic to pathogenic by these influences mediates neuronal and synaptic integrity and, ultimately, cognitive status. *Created with BioRender.com.*

SUMMARY

We have highlighted the current understanding of several major genetic, environmental/lifestyle, and cellular molecular mechanistic pathways associated with vascular and non-VaDs—as well as common mechanisms such as oxidative stress, mitochondrial dysfunction, and neuroinflammation—that together exacerbate neuronal, glial, and vascular cell function in higher-order cognitive brain regions to result in neurodegeneration, synapse loss, and ultimately, cognitive impairment and dementia (**Fig. 1**). Additional potential pathogenic mechanisms, which are likely influenced by these mechanisms, include aberrant intracellular trafficking, especially along endosomal-autophagy-lysosomal and stress pathways,[103,104] imbalances in neurotrophic signaling that favor proapoptotic pathways,[105,106] epigenetic and transcriptional dysregulation,[107,108] and dysbiosis of the gut–brain axis.[109] We posit that disease modification for these devastating disorders requires the development of combinatorial therapies that mitigate these molecular pathway imbalances and promote cellular homeostasis in the aging brain.

ACKNOWLEDGMENTS

The authors acknowledge the following support: NIH P01 AG014449, R01 AG060731, P30 AG072931, and the Saint Mary's Foundation (S.E. Counts); NIH R01 HL137694 and R21 AG074514 (A.M. Dorrance); and NIH R01 AG062217 and the Spectrum Health-MSU Alliance Corporation (M.N. Gordon).

DISCLOSURE

The authors declare no disclosures.

REFERENCES

1. Hinz FI, Geschwind DH. Molecular genetics of neurodegenerative dementias. Cold Spring Harbor Perspect Biol 2017;9(4):a023705.
2. Bird TD. Genetic aspects of Alzheimer disease. Genet Med 2008;10(4):231–9.
3. Genin E, Hannequin D, Wallon D, et al. APOE and Alzheimer disease: a major gene with semi-dominant inheritance. Mol Psychiatry 2011;16(9):903–7.
4. Lambert JC, Heath S, Even G, et al. Genome-wide association study identifies variants at CLU and CR1 associated with Alzheimer's disease. Nat Genet 2009;41(10):1094–9.
5. Hollingworth P, Harold D, Sims R, et al. Common variants at ABCA7, MS4A6A/MS4A4E, EPHA1, CD33 and CD2AP are associated with Alzheimer's disease. Nat Genet 2011;43(5):429–35.
6. Rademakers R, Neumann M, Mackenzie IR. Advances in understanding the molecular basis of frontotemporal dementia. Nat Rev Neurol 2012;8(8):423–34.
7. Van Mossevelde S, Engelborghs S, van der Zee J, et al. Genotype-phenotype links in frontotemporal lobar degeneration. Nat Rev Neurol 2018;14(6):363–78.
8. de Majo MTS, Smith BN, Nishimura AL, et al. ALS-associated missense and nonsense TBK1 mutations can both cause loss of kinase function. Neurobiol Aging 2018;7:266.e1–10.
9. Bernardi L, Tomaino C, Anfossi M, et al. Novel PSEN1 and PGRN mutations in early-onset familial frontotemporal dementia. Neurobiol Aging 2009;30(11): 1825–33.
10. Geiger JT, Ding J, Crain B, et al. Next-generation sequencing reveals substantial genetic contribution to dementia with Lewy bodies. Neurobiol Dis 2016;94: 55–62.
11. Kelley BJ, Haidar W, Boeve BF, et al. Alzheimer disease-like phenotype associated with the c.154delA mutation in progranulin. Arch Neurol 2010;67(2):171–7.
12. Orme T, Hernandez D, Ross OA, et al. Analysis of neurodegenerative disease-causing genes in dementia with Lewy bodies. Acta Neuropathol Commun 2020; 8(1):5.
13. Mishra A, Ferrari R, Heutink P, et al. Gene-based association studies report genetic links for clinical subtypes of frontotemporal dementia. Brain 2017;140(5): 1437–46.
14. Tsuang D, Leverenz JB, Lopez OL, et al. APOE epsilon4 increases risk for dementia in pure synucleinopathies. JAMA Neurol 2013;70(2):223–8.
15. Erkkinen MG, Kim MO, Geschwind MD. Clinical neurology and epidemiology of the major neurodegenerative diseases. Cold Spring Harbor Perspect Biol 2018; 10(4):a033118.
16. Mizuno T, Mizuta I, Watanabe-Hosomi A, et al. Clinical and genetic aspects of CADASIL. Front Aging Neurosci 2020;12:91.
17. Livingston G, Huntley J, Sommerlad A, et al. Dementia prevention, intervention, and care: 2020 report of the Lancet Commission. Lancet 2020;396(10248): 413–46.
18. Iadecola C. The pathobiology of vascular dementia. Neuron 2013;80(4):844–66.
19. Cortes-Canteli M, Iadecola C. Alzheimer's disease and vascular aging: JACC focus seminar. J Am Coll Cardiol 2020;75(8):942–51.

20. Iadecola C, Duering M, Hachinski V, et al. Vascular cognitive impairment and dementia: JACC scientific expert panel. J Am Coll Cardiol 2019;73(25):3326–44.

21. Skrobot OA, Black SE, Chen C, et al. Progress toward standardized diagnosis of vascular cognitive impairment: guidelines from the vascular impairment of cognition classification consensus study. Alzheimer's Demen 2018;14(3): 280–92.

22. Rost NS, Brodtmann A, Pase MP, et al. Post-stroke cognitive impairment and dementia. Circ Res 2022;130(8):1252–71.

23. Hodis JD, Gottesman RF, Windham BG, et al. Association of hypertension according to new american college of cardiology/american heart association blood pressure guidelines with incident dementia in the ARIC study cohort. J Am Heart Assoc 2020;9(22):e017546.

24. Group SMIftSR, Williamson JD, Pajewski NM, et al. Effect of intensive vs standard blood pressure control on probable dementia: a randomized clinical trial. J Am Med Assoc 2019;321(6):553–61.

25. Group SMIftSR, Nasrallah IM, Pajewski NM, et al. Association of intensive vs standard blood pressure control with cerebral white matter lesions. J Am Med Assoc 2019;322(6):524–34.

26. Jennings JR, Muldoon MF, Ryan C, et al. Reduced cerebral blood flow response and compensation among patients with untreated hypertension. Neurology 2005;64(8):1358–65.

27. Longden TA, Dabertrand F, Koide M, et al. Capillary K+-sensing initiates retrograde hyperpolarization to increase local cerebral blood flow. Nat Neurosci 2017;20(5):717–26.

28. Koide M, Harraz OF, Dabertrand F, et al. Differential restoration of functional hyperemia by antihypertensive drug classes in hypertension-related cerebral small vessel disease. J Clin Invest 2021;131(18):e149029.

29. Shih AY, Blinder P, Tsai PS, et al. The smallest stroke: occlusion of one penetrating vessel leads to infarction and a cognitive deficit. Nat Neurosci 2013; 16(1):55–63.

30. Nishimura N, Schaffer CB, Friedman B, et al. Penetrating arterioles are a bottleneck in the perfusion of neocortex. Proc Natl Acad Sci U S A 2007;104(1): 365–70.

31. Cipolla MJ, Li R, Vitullo L. Perivascular innervation of penetrating brain parenchymal arterioles. J Cardiovasc Pharmacol 2004;44(1):1–8.

32. Diaz-Otero JM, Yen T-C, Ahmad A, et al. Transient receptor potential vanilloid 4 channels are important regulators of parenchymal arteriole dilation and cognitive function. Microcirculation 2019;26(6):e12535.

33. Liu L, Guo M, Lv X, et al. Role of transient receptor potential vanilloid 4 in vascular function. Front Mol biosciences 2021;8:677661.

34. Matin N, Fisher C, Lansdell TA, et al. Soluble epoxide hydrolase inhibition improves cognitive function and parenchymal artery dilation in a hypertensive model of chronic cerebral hypoperfusion. Microcirculation 2021;28(1):e12653.

35. Griñán-Ferré C, Codony S, Pujol E, et al. Pharmacological inhibition of soluble epoxide hydrolase as a new therapy for alzheimer's disease. Neurotherapeutics 2020;17(4):1825–35.

36. Iliff JJ, Wang M, Liao Y, et al. A paravascular pathway facilitates CSF flow through the brain parenchyma and the clearance of interstitial solutes, including amyloid β. Sci translational Med 2012;4(147):147ra111.

37. Morris AW, Sharp MM, Albargothy NJ, et al. Vascular basement membranes as pathways for the passage of fluid into and out of the brain. Acta Neuropathol 2016;131(5):725–36.
38. Mortensen KN, Sanggaard S, Mestre H, et al. Impaired glymphatic transport in spontaneously hypertensive rats. J Neurosci 2019;39(32):6365–77.
39. Dugger BN, Dickson DW. Pathology of neurodegenerative diseases. Cold Spring Harb Perspect Biol 2017;9(7):a028035.
40. Matej R, Tesar A, Rusina R. Alzheimer's disease and other neurodegenerative dementias in comorbidity: a clinical and neuropathological overview. Clin Biochem 2019;73:26–31.
41. Mueller RL, Combs B, Alhadidy MM, et al. Tau: a signaling hub protein. Front Mol Neurosci 2021;14:647054.
42. Guerrero-Munoz MJ, Gerson J, Castillo-Carranza DL. Tau oligomers: the toxic player at synapses in alzheimer's disease. Front Cell Neurosci 2015;9:464.
43. Reddy PH, Oliver DM. Amyloid beta and phosphorylated tau-induced defective autophagy and mitophagy in alzheimer's disease. Cells 2019;8(5):488.
44. Mansuroglu Z, Benhelli-Mokrani H, Marcato V, et al. Loss of Tau protein affects the structure, transcription and repair of neuronal pericentromeric heterochromatin. Sci Rep 2016;6:33047.
45. Li S, Jin M, Koeglsperger T, et al. Soluble Abeta oligomers inhibit long-term potentiation through a mechanism involving excessive activation of extrasynaptic NR2B-containing NMDA receptors. J Neurosci 2011;31(18):6627–38.
46. Tolar M, Hey J, Power A, et al. Neurotoxic soluble amyloid oligomers drive alzheimer's pathogenesis and represent a clinically validated target for slowing disease progression. Int J Mol Sci 2021;22(12):6355.
47. Brito-Moreira J, Paula-Lima AC, Bomfim TR, et al. Abeta oligomers induce glutamate release from hippocampal neurons. Curr Alzheimer Res 2011;8(5):552–62.
48. Vandal M, Bourassa P, Calon F. Can insulin signaling pathways be targeted to transport Abeta out of the brain? Front Aging Neurosci 2015;7:114.
49. Koga S, Sekiya H, Kondru N, et al. Neuropathology and molecular diagnosis of Synucleinopathies. Mol neurodegeneration 2021;16(1):83.
50. Jellinger KA. Significance of brain lesions in Parkinson disease dementia and Lewy body dementia. Front Neurol Neurosci 2009;24:114–25.
51. Choi MG, Kim MJ, Kim DG, et al. Sequestration of synaptic proteins by alpha-synuclein aggregates leading to neurotoxicity is inhibited by small peptide. PLoS One 2018;13(4):e0195339.
52. Bernal-Conde LD, Ramos-Acevedo R, Reyes-Hernandez MA, et al. Alpha-synuclein physiology and pathology: a perspective on cellular structures and organelles. Front Neurosci 2019;13:1399.
53. Abeliovich A, Schmitz Y, Farinas I, et al. Mice lacking alpha-synuclein display functional deficits in the nigrostriatal dopamine system. Neuron 2000;25(1):239–52.
54. Teixeira M, Sheta R, Idi W, et al. Alpha-synuclein and the endolysosomal system in Parkinson's disease: guilty by association. Biomolecules 2021;11(9):1333.
55. Keating SS, San Gil R, Swanson MEV, et al. TDP-43 pathology: from noxious assembly to therapeutic removal. Prog Neurobiol 2022;211:102229.
56. Meneses A, Koga S, O'Leary J, et al. TDP-43 pathology in alzheimer's disease. Mol neurodegeneration 2021;16(1):84.
57. Nelson PT, Dickson DW, Trojanowski JQ, et al. Limbic-predominant age-related TDP-43 encephalopathy (LATE): consensus working group report. Brain 2019;142(6):1503–27.

58. Prasad A, Bharathi V, Sivalingam V, et al. Molecular mechanisms of TDP-43 misfolding and pathology in amyotrophic lateral sclerosis. Front Mol Neurosci 2019; 12:25.
59. Butterfield DA, Halliwell B. Oxidative stress, dysfunctional glucose metabolism and Alzheimer disease. Nat Rev Neurosci 2019;20(3):148–60.
60. Galliciotti G, De Jaco A, Sepulveda-Falla D, et al. Role of cellular oxidative stress in dementia. In: Martin CR, Preedy VR, editors. Genetics, neurology, behavior, and diet in dementia: the neuroscience of dementia. Cambridge, MA: Academic Press; 2020. p. 147–61, chap 10.
61. Floyd RA, Hensley K. Oxidative stress in brain aging. Implications for therapeutics of neurodegenerative diseases. Neurobiol Aging 2002;23(5):795–807.
62. Kelly SC, He B, Perez SE, et al. Locus coeruleus cellular and molecular pathology during the progression of Alzheimer's disease. Acta Neuropathol Commun 2017;5(1):8.
63. Smith MA, Nunomura A, Zhu X, et al. Metabolic, metallic, and mitotic sources of oxidative stress in Alzheimer disease. *Antioxid Redox Signal* Fall 2000;2(3): 413–20.
64. Williams TI, Lynn BC, Markesbery WR, et al. Increased levels of 4-hydroxynonenal and acrolein, neurotoxic markers of lipid peroxidation, in the brain in Mild Cognitive Impairment and early Alzheimer's disease. Neurobiol Aging 2005; 27(8):1094–9.
65. Kelly SC, Nelson PT, Counts SE. Pontine arteriolosclerosis and locus coeruleus oxidative stress differentiate resilience from mild cognitive impairment in a clinical pathologic cohort. J Neuropathol Exp Neurol 2021;80(4):325–35.
66. Sharma C, Kim SR. Linking oxidative stress and proteinopathy in alzheimer's disease. Antioxidants (Basel) 2021;10(8):1231.
67. Martinez A, Carmona M, Portero-Otin M, et al. Type-dependent oxidative damage in frontotemporal lobar degeneration: cortical astrocytes are targets of oxidative damage. J Neuropathol Exp Neurol 2008;67(12):1122–36.
68. Esteras N, Rohrer JD, Hardy J, et al. Mitochondrial hyperpolarization in iPSC-derived neurons from patients of FTDP-17 with 10+16 MAPT mutation leads to oxidative stress and neurodegeneration. Redox Biol 2017;12:410–22.
69. Garcia-Esparcia P, Lopez-Gonzalez I, Grau-Rivera O, et al. Dementia with Lewy bodies: molecular pathology in the frontal cortex in typical and rapidly progressive forms. Front Neurol 2017;8:89.
70. Gomez-Tortosa E, Gonzalo I, Newell K, et al. Patterns of protein nitration in dementia with Lewy bodies and striatonigral degeneration. Acta Neuropathol 2002;103(5):495–500.
71. Bosco DA, Fowler DM, Zhang Q, et al. Elevated levels of oxidized cholesterol metabolites in Lewy body disease brains accelerate alpha-synuclein fibrilization. Nat Chem Biol 2006;2(5):249–53.
72. Finkel T. Signal transduction by reactive oxygen species. J Cell Biol 2011; 194(1):7–15.
73. Wang W, Zhao F, Ma X, et al. Mitochondria dysfunction in the pathogenesis of Alzheimer's disease: recent advances. Mol neurodegeneration 2020;15(1):30.
74. Beck JS, Mufson EJ, Counts SE. Evidence for mitochondrial UPR gene activation in familial and sporadic Alzheimer's disease. Curr Alzheimer Res 2015; 13(6):610–4.
75. Choi DH, Lee KH, Kim JH, et al. NADPH oxidase 1, a novel molecular source of ROS in hippocampal neuronal death in vascular dementia. Antioxid Redox Signal 2014;21(4):533–50.

76. Sultana R, Piroddi M, Galli F, et al. Protein levels and activity of some antioxidant enzymes in hippocampus of subjects with amnestic mild cognitive impairment. Neurochem Res 2008;33(12):2540–6.

77. Rinaldi P, Polidori MC, Metastasio A, et al. Plasma antioxidants are similarly depleted in mild cognitive impairment and in Alzheimer's disease. Neurobiol Aging 2003;24(7):915–9.

78. Shukla D, Mandal PK, Tripathi M, et al. Quantitation of in vivo brain glutathione conformers in cingulate cortex among age-matched control, MCI, and AD patients using MEGA-PRESS. Hum Brain Mapp 2020;41(1):194–217.

79. Tonnies E, Trushina E. Oxidative stress, synaptic dysfunction, and alzheimer's disease. J Alzheimers Dis 2017;57(4):1105–21.

80. Uddin MS, Lim LW. Glial cells in Alzheimer's disease: from neuropathological changes to therapeutic implications. Ageing Res Rev 2022;78:101622.

81. McGeer PL, Kawamata T, Walker DG, et al. Microglia in degenerative neurological disease. Glia 1993;7(1):84–92.

82. Boraschi D, Italiani P, Weil S, et al. The family of the interleukin-1 receptors. Immunol Rev 2018;281(1):197–232.

83. Rose-John S. Interleukin-6 signalling in health and disease. F1000Res 2020;9: F1000. Faculty Rev-1013.

84. Gough P, Myles IA. Tumor necrosis factor receptors: pleiotropic signaling complexes and their differential effects. Front Immunol 2020;11:585880.

85. Andrews SJ, Fulton-Howard B, Goate A. Interpretation of risk loci from genome-wide association studies of Alzheimer's disease. Lancet Neurol 2020;19(4): 326–35.

86. Bellenguez C, Kucukali F, Jansen IE, et al. New insights into the genetic etiology of Alzheimer's disease and related dementias. Nat Genet 2022;54(4):412–36.

87. Bright F, Werry EL, Dobson-Stone C, et al. Neuroinflammation in frontotemporal dementia. Nat Rev Neurol 2019;15(9):540–55.

88. Amin J, Erskine D, Donaghy PC, et al. Inflammation in dementia with Lewy bodies. Neurobiol Dis 2022;168:105698.

89. Boche D, Gordon MN. Diversity of transcriptomic microglial phenotypes in aging and Alzheimer's disease. Alzheimers Dement 2022;18(2):360–76.

90. Keren-Shaul H, Spinrad A, Weiner A, et al. A unique microglia type Associated with restricting development of alzheimer's disease. Cell 2017;169(7): 1276–1290 e17.

91. Krasemann S, Madore C, Cialic R, et al. The TREM2-APOE pathway drives the transcriptional phenotype of dysfunctional microglia in neurodegenerative diseases. Immunity 2017;47(3):566–81.

92. Liddelow SA, Guttenplan KA, Clarke LE, et al. Neurotoxic reactive astrocytes are induced by activated microglia. Nature 2017;541(7638):481–7.

93. Salminen A, Ojala J, Kauppinen A, et al. Inflammation in Alzheimer's disease: amyloid-beta oligomers trigger innate immunity defence via pattern recognition receptors. Prog Neurobiol 2009;87(3):181–94.

94. Mossanen Parsi M, Duval C, Ariens RAS. Vascular dementia and crosstalk between the complement and coagulation systems. Front Cardiovasc Med 2021;8: 803169.

95. Jiang H, Burdick D, Glabe CG, et al. beta-Amyloid activates complement by binding to a specific region of the collagen-like domain of the C1q A chain. J Immunol 1994;152(10):5050–9.

96. Tenner AJ, Stevens B, Woodruff TM. New tricks for an ancient system: physiological and pathological roles of complement in the CNS. Mol Immunol 2018; 102:3–13.
97. Hong S, Beja-Glasser VF, Nfonoyim BM, et al. Complement and microglia mediate early synapse loss in Alzheimer mouse models. Science 2016; 352(6286):712–6.
98. Fonseca MI, Ager RR, Chu SH, et al. Treatment with a C5aR antagonist decreases pathology and enhances behavioral performance in murine models of Alzheimer's disease. J Immunol 2009;183(2):1375–83.
99. Shi X, Ohta Y, Liu X, et al. Chronic cerebral hypoperfusion activates the coagulation and complement cascades in alzheimer's disease mice. Neuroscience 2019;416:126–36.
100. Fan R, DeFilippis K, Van Nostrand WE. Induction of complement proteins in a mouse model for cerebral microvascular A beta deposition. J neuroinflammation 2007;4:22.
101. Schrag M, Kirshner H. Neuropsychological effects of cerebral amyloid angiopathy. Curr Neurol Neurosci Rep 2016;16(8):76.
102. Bhatia K, Kindelin A, Nadeem M, et al. Complement C3a receptor (C3aR) mediates vascular dysfunction, hippocampal pathology, and cognitive impairment in a mouse model of VCID. Transl Stroke Res 2022. https://doi.org/10.1007/s12975-022-00993-x.
103. Nixon RA. The role of autophagy in neurodegenerative disease. Nat Med 2013; 19(8):983–97.
104. Koren J 3rd, Jinwal UK, Lee DC, et al. Chaperone signalling complexes in Alzheimer's disease. J Cell Mol Med 2009;13(4):619–30.
105. Fahnestock M, Yu G, Coughlin MD. ProNGF: a neurotrophic or an apoptotic molecule? Prog Brain Res 2004;146:107–10.
106. Counts SE, Mufson EJ. The role of nerve growth factor receptors in cholinergic basal forebrain degeneration in prodromal Alzheimer disease. J Neuropathol Exp Neurol 2005;64(4):263–72.
107. Bernstein AI, Lin Y, Street RC, et al. 5-Hydroxymethylation-associated epigenetic modifiers of Alzheimer's disease modulate Tau-induced neurotoxicity. Hum Mol Genet 2016;25(12):2437–50.
108. Beck JS, Madaj Z, Cheema CT, et al. Co-expression network analysis of frontal cortex during the progression of alzheimer's disease. Cereb Cortex 2022;bhac001.
109. Verhaar BJH, Hendriksen HMA, de Leeuw FA, et al. Gut microbiota composition is related to AD pathology. Front Immunol 2021;12:794519.

Prevention and Treatment of Common Forms of Cognitive Impairment and Dementia

The Role of Vascular Risk Factors in Cognitive Impairment and Dementia and Prospects for Prevention

Simin Mahinrad, MD, PhD[a],*, Farzaneh Sorond, MD, PhD[a],
Philip B. Gorelick, MD, MPH[a]

KEYWORDS

• Vascular risk factors • Cognitive impairment • Dementia • Older adults

KEY POINTS

• Vascular risk factors are precursors to vascular and nonvascular types of dementia.
• Modifiable vascular risk factors represent important targets for mitigating dementia risk among older adults.
• Clinical trials of intensive blood pressure lowering and those using a multidomain approach for the management of vascular risk have provided the most promising results for the preservation of brain health.

INTRODUCTION

Geriatricians and allied care providers are trained in the art of diagnosis and management of health-care problems in older persons. As specialists in the treatment of the elderly, geriatricians are frequently asked to evaluate older persons at risk for cognitive impairment or who may have existent mild cognitive impairment (MCI) or dementia.[1] As part of the diagnostic evaluation, clinicians are searching for reversible or treatable causes of cognitive impairment. Often overlooked is the importance of managing modifiable vascular risks that may negatively influence cognition.[2] Advances in clinical epidemiology have led to a primary care agenda for brain health largely based on the modification of vascular risks for the preservation of cognitive health.[3,4]

This article discusses vascular risks as precursors to both vascular and nonvascular forms of cognitive impairment and dementia, their association with cognitive outcomes, and prospects for prevention.

[a] Department of Neurology, Northwestern University, Feinberg School of Medicine, 625 N. Michigan Avenue, 11th Floor, Suite 1150, Chicago, IL 60611, USA
* Corresponding author.
E-mail address: simin.rad@northwestern.edu

Clin Geriatr Med 39 (2023) 123–134
https://doi.org/10.1016/j.cger.2022.07.007
0749-0690/23/© 2022 Elsevier Inc. All rights reserved.

Vascular Risks as Precursors to both Vascular and Nonvascular Types of Cognitive Impairment and Dementia

Over time we have seen a shift of emphasis in our understanding of cognitive disorders from the failure of cerebral function and cognition attributable to arteriosclerosis and reduction of cerebral blood flow to neurodegenerative mechanisms secondary to Alzheimer disease (AD), with recent shift in focus on vascular risks.[4–7] In fact, it was shown in the early 2000s that the absence of vascular risks was a predictor of healthy survival,[8] and as vascular risks accrued according to the Framingham Stroke Risk Profile score, there was a stepwise loss of total cerebral brain volume accompanied by lower cognitive performance.[9] In addition, vascular risks have been closely linked to both atherosclerosis and AD.[10]

With the publication of additional studies, the importance of vascular risks as potential precursors of the dementias has gained traction,[11–14]and it has become apparent that midlife vascular risks such as hypertension are linked to an elevated risk of cognitive impairment and dementia later in life in both vascular and degenerative types of cognitive disorders. Furthermore, mixed neuropathology may be prevalent in older persons dying with cognitive impairment and dementia.[12,15]

The increasing recognition of the role of vascular risks in defining brain health has resulted in significant initiatives focused on preventing or modifying vascular risks as a target to prevent or slow cognitive impairment and dementia.[2] In a seminal publication from an American Heart Association (AHA)/American Stroke Association workgroup, optimal brain health in adults was defined according to AHA's Life's Simple 7 including 4 ideal health behaviors (nonsmoking, physical activity [PA] at goal levels, healthy diet according to current guidance, and body mass index [BMI] <25 kg/m^2) and 3 ideal health factors (untreated blood pressure [BP] < 120/<80 mm Hg, untreated total cholesterol <200 mg/dL, and fasting glucose <100 mg/dL).[2] Support for a brain health initiative is bolstered by expert assessment of the evidence about potentially modifiable vascular risks by the National Academies of Sciences, Engineering and Medicine (NASEM) and the Lancet Dementia Commission, which are summarized in the "Clinics Care Points" section.[16–18]

Role of Key Vascular Risks

Hypertension

Hypertension has been established as one of the most important risk factors for stroke, with a population attributable risk of up to 50%.[19] Hypertension has also been strongly linked with cognitive impairment and increased risk of dementia beyond symptomatic stroke.[20,21] The Atherosclerosis Risk in Communities was one of the largest population-based studies demonstrating the relationship between midlife hypertension and a 20-year decline in various domains of cognition.[22] Midlife hypertension has been consistently linked with an increased risk of all-cause dementia, AD, and vascular dementia.[20] More recently, the relationship between higher BP levels, even in ranges below hypertension diagnosis guidelines, and worse cognition has been reported. For example, higher cumulative exposure to BP levels from early adulthood to midlife has been associated with worse cognition in midlife.[23,24] However, studies focused on hypertension during late life have often failed to find an association,[20,21] or reported nonlinear relationships where both high and low BP levels were correlated with cognitive decline.[20] Overall, a pattern of consistently raised BP during earlier adulthood to midlife followed by low BP levels in later life seems to negatively impact cognition.[25]

Hypertension is often managed pharmacologically using antihypertensive medications. Although antihypertensive medications result in substantial benefits for cardiovascular morbidity and mortality, their role in improving cognition remains promising at best.[20,26] Results of well-designed, randomized clinical trials (RCTs) assessing the impact of various antihypertensive medications on cognitive outcomes are discussed in "Prospects for Prevention" section.

Diabetes Mellitus

Epidemiologic studies have demonstrated a clear link between diabetes mellitus, primarily type 2 diabetes (T2DM), and adverse cognitive outcomes.[27,28] T2DM is associated with lower performance in several cognitive domains[28] that likely start during the prediabetes stage and progress over time at a rate up to 2 times faster than normal aging.[27] T2DM has also been linked with an increased risk of MCI,[29] all-cause dementia,[30] vascular dementia,[30] and AD.[31] The role of glycemic control—as measured by hemoglobin A1c (HbA1c)—in relation to cognition in T2DM remains unclear. Current evidence suggests either weak associations or evidence of nonlinearity where both low and high HbA1c relate to increased dementia risk in T2DM.[27,28] In contrast to T2DM, type 1 diabetes has been consistently linked with subtle decrements in cognition (or *cognitive decrements*) that likely develop soon after diabetes onset and follow a stable pattern over time or have only a slow rate of progression.[27] Risk factors associated with accelerated cognitive decline in diabetics include comorbid vascular risk factors, microvascular and macrovascular diseases, and depression.[27,28]

Although the link between diabetes mellitus and cognitive dysfunction is clear, the effect of diabetes management in ameliorating dementia risk remains unclear. A Cochrane review on the effect of diabetes treatment on cognition did not find good evidence that any specific diabetes medication, or intensive versus standard glycemic control, prevented or delayed cognitive decline in patients with diabetes.[32]

Obesity/Body Mass Index and Hypercholesterolemia

Obesity and body mass index

Epidemiologic studies have linked obesity to adverse neurocognitive outcomes, although findings are inconsistent across the life course. Generally, midlife obesity has been associated with a higher risk of dementia in later life, whereas late-life obesity has often been inversely associated with neurocognitive outcomes.[33] Pooled estimates from prospective studies suggest that midlife obesity (BMI $\geq$ 30 Kg/m^2), but not overweight (25 < BMI < 30 kg/m^2), confers 1.33 excess risk of dementia in later life.[34] However, late-life obesity and overweight (BMI 23–30 Kg/m^2) have been associated with reduced risk of dementia by 25% and 21%, respectively.[35] At the same time, lower BMI and weight loss in older adults have been associated with an increased risk of dementia.[33] Such findings in older adults have been attributed to several biases, namely reverse causation bias.[33,36] Preclinical weight changes in years before dementia diagnosis has been estimated to result in 10% loss of body weight due to factors such as predementia apathy, loss of initiative, and decreased olfactory function.[37] Therefore, weight loss close to the diagnosis of dementia may underlie the preclinical phase of neurodegeneration.[36,37] Overall, midlife obesity and weight loss in later life seem to characterize the trajectory of BMI as it relates to dementia.[37]

Many RCTs have assessed the effect of weight loss on cognition, although evidence on incident MCI and dementia is lacking. Pooled results from a meta-analysis of 7 RCTs showed that intentional weight loss improves memory over short periods (8–48 weeks).[38]

Hypercholesterolemia

Higher cholesterol levels have been associated with adverse neurocognitive outcomes with inconsistent findings for midlife versus late-life studies. Although cholesterol measured in midlife has been generally linked with increased dementia risk in later life,[39] late-life studies show no or negative correlations.[40] Higher cholesterol levels in midlife followed by declining levels from mid-to-late life may characterize the life-course trajectory of cholesterol as it relates to dementia.[25]

Hypercholesterolemia is often managed pharmacologically using statin medications. Although observational studies have suggested a relationship between statin use and reduced risk of dementia,[26] well-designed RCTs have failed to show cognitive benefit or harm associated with statin use.[41] Therefore, current evidence does not support initiating statins in older adults to prevent cognitive decline but indirect evidence from observational studies may support their use in midlife to reduce dementia risk.[26]

Cigarette Smoking

Evidence from experimental and epidemiologic studies suggests that cigarette smoking is associated with significant neurobiological and neurocognitive abnormalities.[42] Tobacco smoking, especially in midlife, is a risk factor for late-life cognitive decline, all-cause dementia, vascular dementia, and AD.[43,44] Although some early studies suggested a protective effect of smoking on AD risk among the elderly, it has largely proven to be attributed to the bias in observational studies of late-life versus midlife individuals due to survival bias and competing risk of death.[45,46] Moreover, tobacco industry affiliation has been shown to play a significant role in early studies of smoking-related cognitive outcomes.[47] Smoking history has generally not been associated with increased dementia risk[44] but earlier smoking cessation may reduce dementia risk.[48] For example, recent smoking cession (<9 years) was associated with increased risk of dementia, whereas quitting smoking for 9 years or greater was not associated with increased dementia risk.[48]

Physical Activity and Diet

Physical activity

Understanding the impact of PA on brain health is complicated because patterns of PA change according to age, sex, presence of comorbidities, and social and cultural factors.[18,49] Furthermore, baseline cognitive impairment and neurodegeneration could influence mobility, motivation, and goals for engagement in PA, hence, introducing bias in observational studies of PA and dementia risk.[49,50] To date, observational studies suggest that PA may be protective against adverse cognitive outcomes, whereas reverse causation bias cannot be excluded.[49] Overall, in nondemented individuals, high and low-to-moderate levels of PA have been shown to reduce the risk for cognitive decline by 38% and 35% compared with sedentary individuals.[51] Among middle-aged adults, lack of midlife leisure-time PA is associated with a greater incidence of dementia during 14 years.[52]

Pooled results from meta-analyses of RCTs on exercise training concluded that exercise improves cognition in adults aged older than 50 years, including those with MCI.[18] Accordingly, exercise, especially aerobic exercise, may have a small but beneficial impact on cognition in cognitively normal individuals.[26]

Diet

Dietary interventions prevent conditions that increase the risk for dementia, including diabetes and cardiovascular diseases.[26] A direct link between individual dietary components and neurocognitive outcomes has also been demonstrated. Such nutrients include fruits, vegetables, fish, polyunsaturated fatty acids, nuts, olive oil, and coffee.[26,53] However, during the last 5 years, research has moved toward studying overall diet composition and dietary patterns rather than individual dietary components.[53]

Examples of these dietary patterns include the Mediterranean (MEDi) diet, Dietary Approaches to Stop Hypertension (DASH) diet, and Mediterranean-DASH Intervention for Neurodegenerative Delay (MIND) diet. Population-based studies have shown that higher adherence to these dietary patterns is associated with a reduced risk of dementia, AD, and cognitive decline.[53,54]

Meta-analyses of RCTs on dietary interventions found no evidence for dietary supplements to preserve cognition or reduce dementia risk.[18,26] However, a meta-analysis of 5 RCTs found moderate evidence for the beneficial effect of the MEDi diet on global cognition in cognitively normal individuals.[55]

PROSPECTS FOR PREVENTION: WHAT HAVE MAJOR CLINICAL TRIALS AND MULTIDOMAIN INTERVENTIONAL STUDIES TAUGHT US ABOUT VASCULAR RISKS?

Vascular risks are well known to be causal links for stroke, myocardial infarction, heart failure, and other cardiovascular diseases.[2] As such, the treatment or prevention of these factors, at the very least, will reduce the risk of cardiovascular disorders. An additional benefit of modification or prevention of vascular risks may be preserving brain health and preventing cognitive impairment and dementia.[20] In this section, we discuss interventional studies in relation to vascular risks and cognitive outcomes.

Studies Targeting 1 Key Vascular Risk

Systolic Blood Pressure Intervention Trial (SPRINT) and Memory and Cognition in Decreased Hypertension (SPRINT MIND).[56–59]

Systolic Blood Pressure Intervention Trial (SPRINT) tested the effect of intensive systolic BP (SBP) lowering (target goal: <120 mm Hg) versus standard treatment (target goal: <140 mm Hg) on prevention of key cardiovascular outcomes.[56] Memory and Cognition in Decreased Hypertension (SPRINT MIND) is a companion study of SPRINT whereby the intensive SBP lowering strategy was tested among 9361 participants in relation to the primary outcome of probable dementia and the secondary outcomes of MCI and the composite of MCI plus dementia, respectively.[57]

The main primary and secondary cognitive results of SPRINT MIND are listed in **Table 1**. Overall, the primary outcome, probable dementia, was not significantly different between the intensive versus standard treatment groups.[57] However, both secondary cognitive outcomes, MCI and the composite of MCI plus probable dementia, were significantly decreased by intensive BP lowering. In relation to magnetic resonance imaging biomarkers, intensive BP lowering therapy was associated with a smaller increase in cerebral white matter volume but a greater decrease in total brain volume.[58,59] It is important to note that the main phase SPRINT cardiovascular outcome study was stopped prematurely based on results favoring the intensive SBP lowering treatment.[56] As such the primary findings of SPRINT MIND must be considered in the context of a statistically underpowered outcome for probable dementia.

Earlier BP lowering trials did not show a significant positive signal for the preservation of cognition with BP lowering. A marginally beneficial signal for BP lowering on cognition was reported in 2 RCT.[60,61] A review of the individual trials is outside the scope of this article, and reviewed by the authors elsewhere.[20,62] In the Action to Control Cardiovascular Risk in Diabetes Memory in Diabetes (ACCORD MIND) trial, a companion study to ACCORD and similar to SPRINT, but for diabetic patients, there was no difference in relation to the intensive SBP lowering treatment versus standard treatment arm for verbal memory and executive function.[63] Furthermore, there was a statistically significant greater decrease in total brain volume at 40 months for intensive compared with standard SBP treatment.

Table 1 Main findings of SPRINT MIND		
SPRINT MIND Demographics: **Median Age = 67.9 y** **Percent Women Participants = 35.6%**		
Primary Outcome	Secondary Outcome	Brain Imaging Results
Probable dementia: 7.2 vs 8.6 cases per 1000 person-years for intensive vs standard BP lowering HR: 0.83 (95% CI, 0.67–1.04)	MCI: 14.6 vs 18.3 cases per 1000 person-years for intensive vs standard BP lowering HR: 0.81 (95% CI, 0.69–0.95)	a. Intensive BP lowering was associated with a smaller increase in WM volume but a greater decrease in TBV. However, the differences were small
	Composite of MCI + probable dementia: 20.2 vs 24.1 cases per 1000 person-years for intensive vs standard BP lowering HR: 0.85 (95% CI of 0.74–0.97)	b. Intensive BP lowering was associated with a greater decrease in HippV (consistent with the observation of greater decrease in TBV); however, other MRI brain biomarkers of AD were not significantly affected

Abbreviations: BP, blood pressure; CI, confidence interval; HippV: hippocampus volume; HR, hazard ratio; MCI, mild cognitive impairment; TBV, total brain volume; WM, white mater.
Data from Refs.[57–59]

Multidomain Interventions

It is argued that single vascular risk factor interventions may not be adequate to assure the prevention of cognitive impairment or dementia.[20,62] Therefore, it may be advantageous to administer multidomain interventions to modify vascular risks. One such study, Finnish Geriatric Intervention Study to Prevent Cognitive Impairment and Disability (FINGER), targeted diet, exercise, and cognitive training, and vascular risk monitoring, whereas the control group received counseling on general health.[64] The primary outcome was a change in cognition according to a comprehensive neuropsychological test battery (NTB), whereby there were between-group differences in the NTB scores annually of 0.022 (95% CL of 0.002, 0.042; $P = .030$) favoring the multidomain intervention group. In addition to improvement in overall cognition, there were significant benefits on executive function, processing speed, and BMI, dietary habits, and PA.[64] The promising results have led to a FINGERS worldwide network study to determine if the results can be validated in diverse populations. Other multidomain interventional studies are reviewed elsewhere.[62] The latter studies have been less successful in relation to improving cognitive outcomes.

Other Interventions

As previously mentioned, there is insufficient evidence to conclude that the treatment of diabetes mellitus or lipids (eg, statin therapy), or administration of vitamins or other supplements or dietary modification definitively reduces the risk of cognitive impairment or dementia.[16] In addition, there is no high level evidence that administration of low-dose aspirin (100 mg/d) is effective in preventing dementia, MCI, or cognitive decline.[65]

Prospects for Prevention and Practical Guidance for Maintenance of Cognition and Brain Health

Of all the vascular risks, hypertension is the one factor with the largest body of observational epidemiologic and clinical trial study data in the context of brain health.

Disparate and potentially flawed study designs across various RCTs have made it diffi-cult to show a consistent and positive signal in relation to BP lowering and preserva-tion of cognition.[62] However, if one focuses on BP lowering trials of SBP lowering a 10 mm Hg or greater difference compared with the comparison group, it seems that one is more likely to find a beneficial effect of BP lowering on cognition.[66] Furthermore, there does not seem to be a preferred BP lowering medication class for cognitive maintenance suggesting that BP lowering may be the key factor rather than the class of medication.[67] Nonetheless, in a secondary analysis of SPRINT, antihypertensive medications that stimulated type 2 and 4 angiotensin II receptors compared with those that inhibit the receptors were associated with lower rates of incident cognitive impair-ment possibly by promoting beneficial effects on reduced brain ischemia, better blood flow, and improved memory.[68]

SPRINT MIND provides the strongest evidence thus far in relation to intensive SBP lowering for maintenance of cognition, and FINGER provides the most promise for a multidomain approach to vascular risk factor control for preservation of cognition.[57,64] There remain, however, unanswered questions that we have reviewed elsewhere.[20,69] Of note, a recent publication from SPRINT suggests that intensive BP lowering when compared with standard BP lowering was associated with increased rather than decreased cerebral perfusion, especially among those with a history of cardiovascular disease.[70] There is a clear need for additional mechanistic studies in this domain.

Based on the above considerations, we provide the following guidance for BP con-trol for the maintenance of cognition in older persons:[20]

1. It is reasonable to lower BP to prevent cognitive impairment and dementia;[71]
2. The exact BP lowering target to maintain cognitive function remains uncertain; however, for persons who meet SPRINT MIND study eligibility criteria, it may be reasonable to aim for an SBP target of 120 mm Hg and follow SPRINT guidance on which BP lowering medications to administer;
3. For persons who do not meet SPRINT MIND criteria and who can tolerate SBP lowering, it may be reasonable to aim for an SBP target of 130 mm Hg or lesser, a national guidance target in the United States;[71]
4. For persons who have difficulty tolerating BP lowering because of the occurrence of adverse events, it may be reasonable to aim for an SBP target of 130 to 160 mm Hg, by titrating SBP control to the best tolerated SBP level; and
5. Management of other non-BP vascular risks is indicated to promote overall cardio-vascular and possibly brain health.

SUMMARY

Epidemiologic studies have contributed key insights into the association between vascular risk factors and cognitive impairment across the life course. Hypertension is the one factor with the largest body of evidence. Current data suggest that hyper-tension as early as midlife serves as a predictor of cognitive impairment in later life. Midlife exposure to other vascular risk factors, including T2DM, obesity, hypercholes-terolemia, smoking, physical inactivity, and an unhealthy diet, has been consistently linked with cognitive impairment in later life. However, findings from late-life studies have been less consistent, showing weak, nonlinear, or even inverse correlations. These inconsistencies have been attributed to biases inherent in observational studies. Therefore, RCTs provide a more definitive answer on the causal link between vascular risk factors and cognitive outcomes.

As more study data are being accrued, especially in the realm of RCTs, we suggest managing vascular risks according to national or international guidelines for the prevention of stroke and other cardiovascular diseases or preferentially according to those for the maintenance of brain health.[16,17,26] As new high-impact study results are published, practitioners will need to adjust the management of vascular risks according to the new findings. We anticipate that multidomain interventions will be required for preservation of brain health and cognition.

CLINICS CARE POINTS

National Academies of Sciences, Engineering and Medicine (NASEM) Guidance[16]

Encouraging but inconclusive evidence for:
• Blood pressure management for persons with high BP to prevent, delay, or slow AD; and
• Physical activity to delay or slow age-related cognitive decline.

Additional research is needed as insufficient evidence exists for:
• Diabetes mellitus treatment;
• Dietary interventions;
• Lipid lowering therapy (eg, statins); and
• Vitamin B12 plus folic acid supplementation.

Lancet Dementia Commission on Prevention, Intervention, and Care Guidance[18]

Be ambitious about dementia prevention:
• Treat high BP in middle age (45–65 years) and in older persons (>65 years) without dementia to reduce dementia risk;
• Manage the following vascular risks for the potential to delay or prevent dementia cases: manage obesity in midlife, and smoking, physical inactivity, and diabetes mellitus in older persons.

DISCLOSURE

Dr P.B. Gorelick serves on a Data Monitoring Board for a heart failure study clinical trial of LCZ 696 and cognition sponsored by Novartis.

REFERENCES

1. Jongsiriyanyong S, Limpawattana P. Mild cognitive impairment in clinical practice: a review article. Am J Alzheimers Dis Other Demen 2018;33(8):500–7.
2. Gorelick PB, Furie KL, Iadecola C, et al. Defining optimal brain health in adults: a presidential advisory from the American heart association/American stroke association. Stroke 2017;48(10):e284–303.
3. Lazar RM, Howard VJ, Kernan WN, et al. A primary care agenda for brain health: a scientific statement from the American heart association. Stroke 2021;52(6): e295–308.
4. US Department of Health and Human Services. National plan to address Alzheimer's disease: 2021 update 2021. Available at: https://aspe.hhs.gov/reports/national-plan-2021-update. Accessed December 29, 2021.
5. Gorelick PB. Vascular cognitive impairment. In: Lazar RM, Browndyke JN, Pond MA, editors. Neurovascular neuropsychology. 2nd ed. Cham: Springer; 2020. p. 121–38.
6. Gorelick PB, Mangone CA. Vascular dementias in the elderly. Clin Geriatr Med 1991;7(3):599–615.
7. Hachinski V, Einhaupl K, Ganten D, et al. Preventing dementia by preventing stroke: the Berlin Manifesto. Alzheimers Dement 2019;15(7):961–84.

8. Willcox BJ, He Q, Chen R, et al. Midlife risk factors and healthy survival in men. JAMA 2006;296(19):2343–50.
9. Elias MF, Sullivan LM, D'Agostino RB, et al. Framingham stroke risk profile and lowered cognitive performance. Stroke 2004;35(2):404–9.
10. Casserly I, Topol E. Convergence of atherosclerosis and Alzheimer's disease: inflammation, cholesterol, and misfolded proteins. Lancet 2004;363(9415): 1139–46.
11. Gottesman RF, Schneider AL, Zhou Y, et al. Association between midlife vascular risk factors and estimated brain amyloid deposition. JAMA 2017;317(14): 1443–50.
12. Lane CA, Barnes J, Nicholas JM, et al. Associations between vascular risk across adulthood and brain pathology in late life: evidence from a British birth cohort. JAMA Neurol 2020;77(2):175–83.
13. Rabin JS, Klein H, Kirn DR, et al. Associations of physical activity and beta-amyloid with longitudinal cognition and neurodegeneration in clinically normal older adults. JAMA Neurol 2019;76(10):1203–10.
14. Vemuri P, Lesnick TG, Przybelski SA, et al. Age, vascular health, and Alzheimer disease biomarkers in an elderly sample. Ann Neurol 2017;82(5):706–18.
15. Iadecola C, Yaffe K, Biller J, et al. Impact of hypertension on cognitive function: a scientific statement from the American heart association. Hypertension 2016; 68(6):e67–94.
16. National Academies of Sciences E, and medicine; health and medicine division; board on health Sciences policy; committee on preventing dementia and cognitive impairment. In: Downey A, Stroud C, Landis S, et al, editors. Preventing cognitive decline and dementia: a way forward. Washington, DC: National Academies Press (US); 2017.
17. Livingston G, Sommerlad A, Orgeta V, et al. Dementia prevention, intervention, and care. Lancet 2017;390(10113):2673–734.
18. Livingston G, Huntley J, Sommerlad A, et al. Dementia prevention, intervention, and care: 2020 report of the Lancet Commission. Lancet 2020;396(10248): 413–46.
19. Unger T, Borghi C, Charchar F, et al. 2020 International society of hypertension global hypertension practice guidelines. Hypertension 2020;75(6):1334–57.
20. Mahinrad S, Sorond FA, Gorelick PB. Hypertension and cognitive dysfunction: a review of mechanisms, life-course observational studies and clinical trial results. Rev Cardiovasc Med 2021;22(4):1429–49.
21. Iadecola C, Gottesman RF. Neurovascular and cognitive dysfunction in hypertension. Circ Res 2019;124(7):1025–44.
22. Gottesman RF, Schneider AL, Albert M, et al. Midlife hypertension and 20-year cognitive change: the atherosclerosis risk in communities neurocognitive study. JAMA Neurol 2014;71(10):1218–27.
23. Yaffe K, Vittinghoff E, Pletcher MJ, et al. Early adult to midlife cardiovascular risk factors and cognitive function. Circulation 2014;129(15):1560–7.
24. Mahinrad S, Kurian S, Garner CR, et al. Cumulative blood pressure exposure during young adulthood and mobility and cognitive function in midlife. Circulation 2020;141(9):712–24.
25. Peters R, Peters J, Booth A, et al. Trajectory of blood pressure, body mass index, cholesterol and incident dementia: systematic review. Br J Psychiatry 2020; 216(1):16–28.
26. Organization WH. Risk reduction of cognitive decline and dementia. Geneva: WHO guidelines; 2019.

27. Biessels GJ, Despa F. Cognitive decline and dementia in diabetes mellitus: mechanisms and clinical implications. Nat Rev Endocrinol 2018;14(10):591–604.
28. Koekkoek PS, Kappelle LJ, van den Berg E, et al. Cognitive function in patients with diabetes mellitus: guidance for daily care. Lancet Neurol 2015;14(3):329–40.
29. Luchsinger JA, Reitz C, Patel B, et al. Relation of diabetes to mild cognitive impairment. Arch Neurol 2007;64(4):570–5.
30. Gudala K, Bansal D, Schifano F, et al. Diabetes mellitus and risk of dementia: a meta-analysis of prospective observational studies. J Diabetes Investig 2013; 4(6):640–50.
31. Zhang J, Chen C, Hua S, et al. An updated meta-analysis of cohort studies: diabetes and risk of Alzheimer's disease. Diabetes Res Clin Pract 2017;124:41–7.
32. Areosa Sastre A, Vernooij RW, Gonzalez-Colaco Harmand M, et al. Effect of the treatment of Type 2 diabetes mellitus on the development of cognitive impairment and dementia. Cochrane Database Syst Rev 2017;6:CD003804.
33. Brenowitz WD. Invited commentary: body mass index and risk of dementia-potential Explanations for life-course differences in risk estimates and Future research directions. Am J Epidemiol 2021;190(12):2511–4.
34. Albanese E, Launer LJ, Egger M, et al. Body mass index in midlife and dementia: systematic review and meta-regression analysis of 589,649 men and women followed in longitudinal studies. Alzheimers Dement (Amst) 2017;8:165–78.
35. Qu Y, Hu HY, Ou YN, et al. Association of body mass index with risk of cognitive impairment and dementia: a systematic review and meta-analysis of prospective studies. Neurosci Biobehav Rev 2020;115:189–98.
36. Kivimaki M, Luukkonen R, Batty GD, et al. Body mass index and risk of dementia: analysis of individual-level data from 1.3 million individuals. Alzheimers Dement 2018;14(5):601–9.
37. Singh-Manoux A, Dugravot A, Shipley M, et al. Obesity trajectories and risk of dementia: 28 years of follow-up in the Whitehall II Study. Alzheimers Dement 2018; 14(2):178–86.
38. Veronese N, Facchini S, Stubbs B, et al. Weight loss is associated with improvements in cognitive function among overweight and obese people: a systematic review and meta-analysis. Neurosci Biobehav Rev 2017;72:87–94.
39. Power MC, Rawlings A, Sharrett AR, et al. Association of midlife lipids with 20-year cognitive change: a cohort study. Alzheimers Dement 2018;14(2):167–77.
40. Anstey KJ, Ashby-Mitchell K, Peters R. Updating the evidence on the association between serum cholesterol and risk of late-life dementia: review and meta-analysis. J Alzheimers Dis 2017;56(1):215–28.
41. Bunt CW, Hogan AJ. The effect of statins on dementia and cognitive decline. Am Fam Physician 2017;95(3):151–2.
42. Durazzo TC, Mattsson N, Weiner MW. Alzheimer's Disease Neuroimaging I. Smoking and increased Alzheimer's disease risk: a review of potential mechanisms. Alzheimers Dement 2014;10(3 Suppl):S122–45.
43. Sabia S, Elbaz A, Dugravot A, et al. Impact of smoking on cognitive decline in early old age: the Whitehall II cohort study. Arch Gen Psychiatry 2012;69(6): 627–35.
44. Zhong G, Wang Y, Zhang Y, et al. Smoking is associated with an increased risk of dementia: a meta-analysis of prospective cohort studies with investigation of potential effect modifiers. PLoS One 2015;10(3):e0118333.
45. Chang CC, Zhao Y, Lee CW, et al. Smoking, death, and Alzheimer disease: a case of competing risks. Alzheimer Dis Assoc Disord 2012;26(4):300–6.

46. Weuve J, Tchetgen Tchetgen EJ, Glymour MM, et al. Accounting for bias due to selective attrition: the example of smoking and cognitive decline. Epidemiology 2012;23(1):119–28.

47. Cataldo JK, Prochaska JJ, Glantz SA. Cigarette smoking is a risk factor for Alzheimer's Disease: an analysis controlling for tobacco industry affiliation. J Alzheimers Dis 2010;19(2):465–80.

48. Deal JA, Power MC, Palta P, et al. Relationship of cigarette smoking and time of quitting with incident dementia and cognitive decline. J Am Geriatr Soc 2020; 68(2):337–45.

49. Erickson KI, Donofry SD, Sewell KR, et al. Cognitive aging and the promise of physical activity. Annu Rev Clin Psychol 2022;18:417–42.

50. Kivimaki M, Singh-Manoux A, Pentti J, et al. Physical inactivity, cardiometabolic disease, and risk of dementia: an individual-participant meta-analysis. BMJ 2019;365:l1495.

51. Sofi F, Valecchi D, Bacci D, et al. Physical activity and risk of cognitive decline: a meta-analysis of prospective studies. J Intern Med 2011;269(1):107–17.

52. Palta P, Sharrett AR, Deal JA, et al. Leisure-time physical activity sustained since midlife and preservation of cognitive function: the Atherosclerosis Risk in Communities Study. Alzheimers Dement 2019;15(2):273–81.

53. Pistollato F, Iglesias RC, Ruiz R, et al. Nutritional patterns associated with the maintenance of neurocognitive functions and the risk of dementia and Alzheimer's disease: a focus on human studies. Pharmacol Res 2018;131:32–43.

54. Jennings A, Cunnane SC, Minihane AM. Can nutrition support healthy cognitive ageing and reduce dementia risk? BMJ 2020;369:m2269.

55. Radd-Vagenas S, Duffy SL, Naismith SL, et al. Effect of the Mediterranean diet on cognition and brain morphology and function: a systematic review of randomized controlled trials. Am J Clin Nutr 2018;107(3):389–404.

56. Group SR, Lewis CE, Fine LJ, et al. Final report of a trial of intensive versus standard blood-pressure control. N Engl J Med 2021;384(20):1921–30.

57. Group SMIftSR, Williamson JD, Pajewski NM, et al. Effect of intensive vs standard blood pressure control on probable dementia: a randomized clinical trial. JAMA 2019;321(6):553–61.

58. Group SMIftSR, Nasrallah IM, Pajewski NM, et al. Association of intensive vs standard blood pressure control with cerebral white matter lesions. JAMA 2019; 322(6):524–34.

59. Nasrallah IM, Gaussoin SA, Pomponio R, et al. Association of intensive vs standard blood pressure control with magnetic resonance imaging biomarkers of alzheimer disease: secondary analysis of the SPRINT MIND randomized trial. JAMA Neurol 2021;78(5):568–77.

60. Forette F, Seux ML, Staessen JA, et al. The prevention of dementia with antihypertensive treatment: new evidence from the Systolic Hypertension in Europe (Syst-Eur) study. Arch Intern Med 2002;162(18):2046–52.

61. Tzourio C, Anderson C, Chapman N, et al. Effects of blood pressure lowering with perindopril and indapamide therapy on dementia and cognitive decline in patients with cerebrovascular disease. Arch Intern Med 2003;163(9):1069–75.

62. Gorelick PB. Prevention of cognitive impairment: scientific guidance and windows of opportunity. J Neurochem 2018;144(5):609–16.

63. Williamson JD, Launer LJ, Bryan RN, et al. Cognitive function and brain structure in persons with type 2 diabetes mellitus after intensive lowering of blood pressure and lipid levels: a randomized clinical trial. JAMA Intern Med 2014;174(3): 324–33.

64. Ngandu T, Lehtisalo J, Solomon A, et al. A 2 year multidomain intervention of diet, exercise, cognitive training, and vascular risk monitoring versus control to prevent cognitive decline in at-risk elderly people (FINGER): a randomised controlled trial. Lancet 2015;385(9984):2255–63.

65. Ryan J, Storey E, Murray AM, et al. Randomized placebo-controlled trial of the effects of aspirin on dementia and cognitive decline. Neurology 2020;95(3): e320–31.

66. Peters R, Warwick J, Anstey KJ, et al. Blood pressure and dementia: what the SPRINT-MIND trial adds and what we still need to know. Neurology 2019; 92(21):1017–8.

67. Peters R, Yasar S, Anderson CS, et al. Investigation of antihypertensive class, dementia, and cognitive decline: a meta-analysis. Neurology 2020;94(3):e267–81.

68. Marcum ZA, Cohen JB, Zhang C, et al. Association of antihypertensives that stimulate vs inhibit types 2 and 4 angiotensin II receptors with cognitive impairment. JAMA Netw Open 2022;5(1):e2145319.

69. Gorelick PB, Sorond F. Cognitive function in SPRINT: where do we go next? Lancet Neurol 2020;19(11):880–1.

70. Dolui S, Detre JA, Gaussoin SA, et al. Association of intensive vs standard blood pressure control with cerebral blood flow: secondary analysis of the SPRINT MIND randomized clinical trial. JAMA Neurol 2022;79(4):380–9.

71. Gorelick PB, Whelton PK, Sorond F, et al. Blood pressure management in stroke. Hypertension 2020;76(6):1688–95.

Treatment of Vascular and Neurodegenerative Forms of Cognitive Impairment and Dementias

Landon Perlett, MD, Clinical Fellow in Neurology,
Eric E. Smith, MD, MPH, Professor of Neurology*

KEYWORDS

• Alzheimer disease • Dementia • Treatment • Cognition

KEY POINTS

• Cognitive-enhancing medications, the cholinesterase inhibitors and memantine, are indicated for dementia caused by some types of neurodegenerative diseases including Alzheimer disease.
• Identifying and treating vascular risk factors may slow the rate of cognitive decline.
• Advance care planning, enhancing safety (including ability to drive), and providing home care services can increase quality of life and extend the time spent living in the community.

INTRODUCTION

The treatment of dementia has been evolving, although slowly, during the last few decades. Pharmacotherapeutic options remain limited to just a few medications, although there is hope that further research into targeted monoclonal antibodies (mAbs) may deliver new therapies for neurodegenerative diseases. As we are now able to diagnose dementia subtypes earlier by means of PET imaging or cerebrospinal fluid (CSF) biomarkers, novel treatments targeting selected patient populations have a better chance of success than we have previously known.

Because of the absence of disease-modifying therapies (DMTs), the focus of management remains on symptomatic treatments for cognition and memory. Additionally, there are many options to target other sequelae of dementia such as neuropsychiatric symptoms, as well as the hope that better cardiovascular risk factor reduction may prevent cognitive decline and that physical, social, and cognitive therapies may

Department of Clinical Neurosciences, University of Calgary, Calgary, Alberta, Canada
* Corresponding author. Room 2941 Health Sciences Centre, 3330 Hospital Drive Northwest, Calgary, Alberta T2N 4N1, Canada.
E-mail address: eesmith@ucalgary.ca

Clin Geriatr Med 39 (2023) 135–149
https://doi.org/10.1016/j.cger.2022.07.008
0749-0690/23/© 2022 Elsevier Inc. All rights reserved.

enhance cognitive reserve. Addressing auditory and visual impairments may also improve cognition.

Another important aspect of care is to optimize support for living safely with good quality of life and to support the health of informal caregivers. This includes discussions around advanced care planning, as well as assessment of other safety concerns including the risk of falls, access to firearms, and driving safety.

The aim of this article is to review the pharmacotherapies available today, as well as those emerging in research trials, and to briefly list the principles of nonpharmacological management. An overview of patient-centered dementia care is shown in **Fig. 1**.

COGNITIVE-ENHANCING MEDICATIONS FOR NEURODEGENERATIVE DISEASES

Without any proven DMTs for neurodegenerative diseases, symptomatic medications are foundational to dementia treatment. There are currently 3 cholinesterase inhibitors (ChE-I) broadly available, as well as one N-methyl-D-aspartate (NMDA) receptor antagonist. Memantine was the last medication approved for the treatment of dementia by the Food and Drug Administration (FDA) in 2003, and there have been no new medications approved in nearly 2 decades.[1] Selection of a particular medication depends on a variety of factors including dementia type and stage of severity, ease of administration, tolerability, insurance coverage or cost, and is typically decided on an individual case basis.[2]

Cholinesterase Inhibitors

There are currently 3 different ChE-Is available: donepezil, rivastigmine, and galantamine. The efficacy profiles of each medication are similar across several meta-analyses,[3,4] and the selection of a specific medication is typically chosen based on other factors such as dosage frequency or tolerability.[2] An overview is shown in **Table 1**.

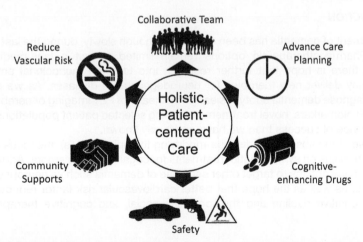

Fig. 1. Overview of Dementia Care. Collaborative team may include allied health professionals such as social workers, neuropsychologists, and occupational therapists. Advance care planning should include designation of an enduring power of attorney, will, and advance medical directives. Cognitive-enhancing drugs are summarized in **Table 1**. Safety should include assessment of driving, access to firearms, risk for falls, and wandering. Community supports may include home care programs, day programs, and support from community-based charitable organizations. Vascular risk factors should be identified and treated.

Table 1
Cognitive-enhancing mediations for Alzheimer disease and Parkinson disease dementia

Medication	Initial Dose	Maximum Dose	Indication	Mechanisms of Action	Unique Features
Donepezil	5 mg OD	10 mg OD (23 mg tablet available in the United States)	Mild-to-severe AD	Acetylcholinesterase inhibitor	The only ChE-I approved for all stages of AD
Rivastigmine	1.5 mg bid	6 mg bid	Mild-to-moderate AD Mild-to-moderate PDD	Acetylcholinesterase inhibitor Butyrylcholinesterase inhibitor	Available in a dermal patch
Galantamine	4 mg bid	12 mg bid	Mild-to-moderate AD	Acetylcholinesterase inhibitor Possible nicotinic acetylcholine receptor modulator	Available in an extended-release formulation
Memantine	5 mg OD	10 mg bid	Moderate-to-severe AD	NMDA receptor blocker	Best tolerability over the ChE-Is

ChE-Is are reversible inhibitors of cholinesterase, preventing break down of acetyl-choline in the central nervous system. Cholinergic deficits are implicated in some forms of dementia, and as cholinergic neurons are lost, this leads to worsening memory and cognitive function.[5] By stabilizing cholinergic function, modest improvements in cognition and behavioral symptoms are achieved while also temporarily delaying disease progression.[6,7]

ChE-Is are a viable treatment option for Alzheimer disease (AD) as well as Parkinson disease dementias (PDDs). Given how commonly cerebrovascular disease is accompanied by AD pathology, with data showing up to an 84% overlap, treatment with a ChE-I is reasonable in the setting of vascular cognitive impairment (VCI), although they are not labeled by the US FDA for that purpose.[8] When used for Lewy Body dementia (LBD), ChE-Is seem to improve cognition and activities of daily living (ADL), without appearing to worsen motor function.[9] There is insufficient evidence to support their use in other settings, such as mild cognitive impairment (MCI) or frontotemporal dementia variants.[10,11]

Donepezil

The oldest of the current ChE-Is, it is unique in that is approved by the US FDA for use in all stages of AD, from mild to severe.[12] Advantages include a long half-life with once daily dosing, minimal drug–drug interaction profile, and excellent drug absorption.[6] Dosing starts at 5 mg daily and can be increased to 10 mg after a period of 4 to 6 weeks.[13] In 2010, a 23-mg tablet was patented to target advanced AD. The initial trial was somewhat controversial with cognitive benefit only found in post hoc analysis, and further trials showed modest cognitive benefit in severe AD with increasing risk of adverse side effects at higher dosage.[12,14,15]

Rivastigmine

The US FDA approved rivastigmine for use in mild-to-moderate AD as well as mild-to-moderate PDD, and it is sometimes used off-label in LBD. Dosage begins at 1.5 mg twice daily and can be slowly titrated up to 6 mg twice daily as tolerated.[16] Rivastigmine is the only ChE-I available in a transdermal patch, which may be preferred in the setting of dysphagia or suspected medication noncompliance. It also seems to be better tolerated than the oral formulation.[17] Patients require education on patch placement in order to avoid skin reactions or risk of toxicity should multiple patches be applied in error.[18] Finally, rivastigmine is the only drug that also inhibits butyrylcholinesterase (BChE), another enzyme that breaks down acetylcholine. The role that BChE plays in neurodegenerative disease is not yet clear, and further study is warranted.[19]

Galantamine

The last ChE-I to be approved by the US FDA, galantamine is indicated for use in mild-to-moderate AD. It is initiated at 4 mg twice daily, increasing by 8 mg every 4 weeks to max dosage of 12 mg twice a day. An extended-release formulation is also available for once daily dosing.[20,21] It has also been described as a nicotinic ACh receptor modulator as a secondary mechanism of action, although this has recently been questioned.[22] A prodrug of galantamine, gln-1062, has been suggested to have better CNS penetration as well as reduced side effect profile.[23] An intranasal formulation was recently trialed in a small study but further research is still needed.

Memantine

As the only NMDA receptor antagonist drug approved for the treatment of moderate-to-severe AD, it is often used in combination with other ChE-Is in the later stages of disease. The initial dose is 5 mg daily, and 5 mg can be added each week at twice daily dosing to a maximum 10 mg twice a day.[24,25] Unlike the ChE-Is, memantine maintains the highest tolerability profile at the highest dosage, whether used alone or in combination therapy. When used in combination, memantine and donepezil seemed to show the best cognitive response as well as overall cost effectiveness.[26] Interestingly, one randomized controlled trial (RCT) demonstrated diminished efficacy of galantamine and memantine as a combination therapy when compared with galantamine alone, and although the underlying reason was not clear, it was posited that this may be due to memantine's antagonism of nicotinic receptors that had been enhanced by galantamine.[27] In addition, 2 RCTs have demonstrated improvement in cognition in mild-to-moderate VCI when compared with placebo and were well tolerated in that population.[28,29]

Efficacy, Tolerability, and Duration of Therapy of Cognitive-Enhancing Medications

There are few head-to-head studies between ChE-Is but several meta-analyses during the last 20 years have shown similar efficacy profiles for improved cognition between all 3 medications.[4,30,31] Data demonstrating improvement of neuropsychiatric symptoms in dementia have been conflicting, although there is suggestion of modest benefit, particularly in combination therapy with memantine.[32] Given the comparative benefits, initial selection of a particular ChE-I can be made on other factors, such as dosage frequency or cost.

The side effect profile is also similar between ChE-Is. The most common side effects are gastrointestinal (nausea, diarrhea, anorexia), although cardiovascular (bradycardia and arrhythmias) and neurologic (dizziness, headache, insomnia) symptoms are seen.[33] Of the ChE-Is, donepezil seems to have the lowest rate of discontinuation and risk of adverse events, whereas rivastigmine was associated with the highest risk of adverse events.[4,26] Memantine is the best tolerated of all, with a comparable safety profile to placebo.[34] Once an agent has been chosen, it should be continued for at least 6 months to monitor for benefit. If no benefit is seen, or the medication is not tolerated, it is reasonable to switch to a different ChE-I. However, if improvement is achieved and then wanes over time, switching to another agent is not recommended.[35]

The total duration of therapy remains unclear because most clinical trials were only 6 to 12 months in duration and clinical guidelines are variable. The AD2000 trial detected a persistent cognitive benefit with donepezil during a period of 2 to 4 years.[36] Post hoc analysis in the DOMINO-AD trial also suggested increased risk of nursing home placement in the following 12 months after donepezil withdrawal.[37] Discontinuation of therapy can be considered if a patient on therapy for more than 12 months continues to decline cognitively with or without previous benefit, if the patient enters end stage dementia, or if a patient develops intolerable side effects.[38]

Emerging Evidence for Antiamyloid Beta Monoclonal Antibodies

In the long search for DMTs for AD, mAbs targeting amyloid-beta may be the most promising approach, but not without controversy. In the setting of AD, several mAbs have been developed and are theorized to either bind amyloid proteins for phagocytosis by macrophages, to enhance the efflux of amyloid beta outside of the blood–brain barrier, or both.

Initial trials of gantenerumab and solanezumab did not find clinical benefit.[39,40] Based on evidence from 2 phase 3 trials, the US FDA granted accelerated approval for aducanumab, an anti-beta amyloid mAb, on the basis that it was proven to reduce signal on amyloid PET scans. This was the first DMT approved for AD, as well as the newest dementia medication in more than 20 years. However, the clinical effectiveness of the drug has been questioned. Evidence for reduced functional decline emerged only after post hoc analysis of the 2 trials, which were originally terminated early due to evidence of futility.[41]

Concern over widespread use of aducanumab has been heightened by its association with amyloid-related imaging abnormalities, consisting of either vasogenic edema or intracranial hemorrhage.[42] The European Medicines Agency declined to authorize aducanumab for treatment of AD, and US Medicare decided to cover the costs of aducanumab only when it is used in clinical trials.[43,44] Currently, there seems to be little use of aducanumab in routine clinical practice in the United States. In the coming years, additional trials of aducanumab and similar antibodies such as donanemab[45] may clarify whether they will play a role in the management of early AD.

TREATMENT OF VASCULAR COGNITIVE IMPAIRMENT AND THE ROLE OF VASCULAR RISK REDUCTION

Cerebrovascular pathology is present in the brain of most persons who die of dementia, often accompanying neurodegenerative pathologic conditions such as AD. In contrast to the neurodegenerative diseases where there is not yet definitive evidence for DMTs, it is known that vascular risk factors can be reduced, and stroke can be prevented. Therefore, targeting vascular risk is currently the most promising method for preventing cognitive decline and preserving cognition. Vascular risk should be assessed, and risk should be reduced in all patients with dementia, including those diagnosed clinically with neurodegenerative causes as well as those with VCI.

Cognitive-Enhancing Medications in Vascular Cognitive Impairment

There are currently no specific pharmacologic interventions indicated by the US FDA for the treatment of cognition in the setting of VCI. Meta-analyses of ChE-Is and memantine for VCI found modest cognitive benefit for donepezil, galantamine, and memantine but treatment came at a cost of side effects; therefore, their role in the treatment of VCI has been controversial.[46,47] Their use in selected patients may be reasonable, with the strongest rationale for treating patients with VCI that have gradually progressive decline and who may also have concomitant AD pathology.[48]

Aspirin

In the ASPREE trial, use of aspirin in the general elderly population did not reduce the incidence of dementia or MCI.[49] When trialed in patients with AD, aspirin did not improve cognitive outcomes and was associated with increased bleeding.[50] For patients with VCI with covert brain infarcts but no history of symptomatic stroke, the use of aspirin may be reasonable but there is no definitive evidence from clinical trials to indicate the effectiveness of this approach.[48] We recommend against using aspirin for patients with only white matter lesions because the pathogenesis of white matter lesions is uncertain and because an increased risk of intracranial bleeding was seen in one small trial.[51]

Control of Vascular Risk Factors

The primary focus of management in VCI should be on cardiovascular risk reduction and stroke prevention, with management of blood pressure, diabetes, dyslipidemia, and obesity, as well as reduction in smoking and alcohol use. For patients with VCI after a prior stroke, preventing the next stroke is the most important objective.

Given that cerebrovascular disease frequently accompanies neurodegenerative diseases, and that so many vascular risk factors are also risk factors for dementia, there should be a focus on vascular risk reduction for all patients with cognitive impairment (MCI or dementia) of any apparent cause. The American Heart Association provides guidance on primary prevention of stroke, which is applicable to all patients with dementia.[52] An earlier article in this issue reviews vascular risk reduction for dementia prevention in greater detail.

COGNITIVE TRAINING

Based in theories of cognitive reserve and neuroplasticity, various nonpharmacologic cognitive-enhancing strategies have been assessed in dementia patients.[53] Research began in the 1980s with pen and paper testing, expanding to computer programs in the 1990s, and now with smart phone and tablet programs. As technology continues to evolve, more therapies are adapting the use of augmented and virtual reality, video games, or electroceutical interventions such as transcranial magnetic stimulation.[54] These interventions rely on the assumption that by performing isolated tasks designed to stimulate a specific cognitive function (ie, verbal memory, logic, and planning), benefit can then be adapted to real-world situations, a concept known as far transfer.[55]

There are 3 main methods used: cognitive stimulation (CS), cognitive rehabilitation (CR), and cognitive training (CT). CS are nonspecific exercises that are usually done in a group setting to enhance cognition and socialization. CR is usually done in a one-on-one setting with the aim of improving a specific deficit such as speech or visual processing. Finally, CT can be done individually or in groups with the intention of improving a specific function such as memory or attention.[56]

Given the heterogeneity of different cognitive interventions that have been studied, it is difficult to systematically evaluate their overall benefits. A recent Cochrane review of 33 trials in those with mild-to-moderate dementia suggested small improvements in global cognition and verbal memory but with low quality of evidence and high risk of bias.[56] A meta-analysis of computerized CT found moderate and significant improvement in measures of global cognition, verbal and nonverbal learning, both verbal and working memory, attention, and psychosocial functioning in those with MCI. However, this was not demonstrated in those with suspected dementia.[57]

At this time, the best evidence for CT in improving cognition and delaying dementia is seen in healthy older individuals and MCI populations. More information on cognitive reserve and CT for dementia can be found in another article in this issue.

MANAGEMENT OF NEUROPSYCHIATRIC SYMPTOMS

Most persons with dementia, up to 98%, will experience neuropsychiatric symptoms, especially in the later stages of disease.[58] Behavioral and psychological symptoms of dementia (BPSD) vary and can manifest as agitation, depression, sleep disorders, hallucinations, or delusions.[59] Later life emergence of persistent neuropsychiatric symptoms, known as mild behavioral impairment, can be predictive of developing cognitive decline and dementia.[60] The presence of these symptoms can affect both the patient and their caregiver(s), resulting in worsening cognitive decline, prolonged hospital stays, and earlier institutionalization.[61]

Selection of a specific agent to manage BPSD should be done carefully because many of these medications are associated with the risk of worsening cognition, falls, or adverse cardiovascular events.[62] Antipsychotics seem to increase mortality in dementia, and this has led to warnings to providers of these drugs in several countries.[63] Drugs for BPSD should be initiated with a "low and slow" methodology and the patient closely monitored for symptomatic benefit or adverse effects. However, nonpharmacological approaches should be the first line of treatment and may include interventions such as occupational therapy, art therapy, and psychological therapy. The management of neurobehavioral and psychiatric disturbances in dementia is covered in greater detail in another article in this issue.

MANAGING SAFETY CONCERNS
Wandering and Pacing

Wandering is a common symptom seen in patients with dementia and is a seemingly aimless or disoriented ambulation, also characterized as lapping or pacing. This behavior can lead to patients becoming lost, cause injuries due to falls, or result in fatigue, weight loss, and earlier institutionalization.[64] Treatment can be challenging. Medications such as ChE-Is, SSRIs, or atypical antipsychotics have been tried. Nonpharmacologic interventions may include exercise or music therapy, personal tracking devices, or camouflaging doorways to reduce elopement.[65]

Falls

Although falls in elderly patients are common, those with cognitive impairment are twice as likely to fall and are 5 times more likely to be admitted to institutional care. Falls may also result in injury such as fractures and concussions.[66] The first step is to review patients for evidence of orthostatic hypotension or visual impairment, as well as any contributing medications such as antipsychotics or benzodiazepines.[67] Although encouraging physical activity is advisable, it is unclear as to which exercises are recommended to reduce the risk of falling.[68,69] Other safety precautions could include the use of hip protectors and low impact flooring, although poor compliance and costs may prohibit their implementation.[70]

Driving Safety

Patients with dementia have a higher risk of becoming involved in a traffic accident when compared with those without. Although people with neurodegenerative cognitive impairment may be capable of driving for some time, given the progressive nature of their disease, it is reasonable to review their driving ability every 6 to 9 months.[71] Evaluation of driving safety can be difficult and varies widely in practice. Asking informants about any recent accidents or traffic violations, as well as their perspective on the safety of the patient's driving, can be helpful.[72] Safe driving correlates with several cognitive domains including visuoconstructional, visuospatial, attention, and executive functioning. Although no single cognitive test can predict driving safety in isolation, some tools that may be helpful include both Trail Making Tests A and B, Symbol Digit Modality Test, clock drawing, as well as intersecting pentagon figure copying.[71,73] Discussion of safe driving in the setting of dementia should be done early in the disease course, and if any concerns are identified then driving cessation or on-road testing is warranted.[74]

Firearm Safety

Around 20% of home caregivers experience aggression or violence from those with dementia, and the presence of a gun in the home adds another layer of risk.[75] People diagnosed with dementia may have an increased risk of suicide, and accessibility to a gun increases that risk.[76] If a firearm is accessible, care providers should ask about the "5 Ls": is the gun loaded, is it locked, are there little children in the home, is the patient feeling *low*, and has the patient properly *learned* how to use the weapon.[77] Although rules regarding firearm possession in those with dementia varies by location, discussion and education of gun safety with patients and caregivers is important in reducing risks to them and society at large.

SUPPORTING QUALITY OF LIFE AND ADVANCED CARE PLANNING
Advanced Care Planning

Given that informed capacity and decision-making will probably be lost as cognition declines, discussions around care planning should happen early and be revisited as patient needs change over time. These discussions should include not only medical care but also estate and financial planning, includinng designation of an enduring power of attorney.[78] Unfortunately, advanced care planning in those with dementia is often neglected and only hoccurs in an estimated 3% to 39% worldwide.[79] Because it is a sensitive topic, approaching it in an individual, patient-centered way is advisable.[80] Advanced care planning increases satisfaction of care for both patients and their caregivers, and may reduce rates of hospitalization or stress for families who find themselves making emergent decisions on behalf of their loved ones.[81] Provision of educational materials on these documents at clinic visits and referral to social work can help families navigate the complexities unique to their situation and respective legal systems.

Community Resources

Most dementia care is provided by informal caregivers, typically spouses or other family members. Caregiver burnout increases with worsening disease severity, particularly when BPSD symptoms are present, such as aggression or delusions, and can result in increased rates of depression and hypertension in caregivers.[82]

Support groups are a great resource for caregivers and have been shown to be effective in reducing stress, depression, and feelings of resentment, as well as improving handling skills and quality of life.[83] Adult day programs can also mitigate caregiver burnout by providing respite, reducing patient behavioral symptoms, and keeping patients engaged in their community who would otherwise be isolated.[84] Other resources that could be explored include speech therapy for those with aphasia or dysarthria, and occupational and physical therapy for those with motor impairment and poor balance.[85–87] Nonprofit organizations—such as the Alzheimer's Association (USA), Alzheimer's Society of Canada, and Alzheimer's Society (UK)—may be able to provide additional services and support.

SUMMARY

Given the lack of DMTs in dementia, a holistic and patient-centered approach is required to provide the excellent care that patients deserve. As these patients are mainly elderly and likely to have other comorbidities, medication reconciliation is pertinent to reduce possible offending drugs, and introduction of new medications should be done slowly and in a supervised fashion to ensure treatment goals are attained. Vascular risk factors should be identified and treated in all patients. Patient and caregiver education and support can allow persons with dementia to live independently in their communities for longer. New therapeutics are emerging that may in the future provide new tools to modify the course of AD and enhance cognition.

CLINICS CARE POINTS

- Cognitive-enhancing medications, including the cholinesterase inhibitors and memantine, are indicated for AD and PDD, with moderate-quality evidence for vascular dementia and LBD.

- There is hope that the course of AD can be modified by monoclonal antibodies that target amyloid beta, although further clinical trials are needed.

- Vascular risk factors should be identified and treated in all patients.

- Multidisciplinary care should include identifying and treating neuropsychiatric symptoms, offering cognitively stimulating activities, planning in advance for loss of capacity to make decisions, and supporting safe living in the community.

DISCLOSURE

Dr L. Perlett reports no conflicts of interest. Dr E.E. Smith reports research grants from the Canadian Institutes of Health Research, and consulting for Eli Lilly.

REFERENCES

1. Areosa SA, Sherriff F, McShane R. Memantine for dementia. Cochrane Database Syst Rev 2005;(2):CD003154.
2. Graham L. AAFP and ACP release guideline on dementia treatment. Am Fam Physician 2008;77(8):1173–5.
3. Birks J. Cholinesterase inhibitors for Alzheimer's disease. Cochrane Database Syst Rev 2006;2006(1):CD005593.
4. Kobayashi H, Ohnishi T, Nakagawa R, et al. The comparative efficacy and safety of cholinesterase inhibitors in patients with mild-to-moderate Alzheimer's disease: a Bayesian network meta-analysis. Int J Geriatr Psychiatry 2016;31(8):892–904.
5. Bartus RT, Dean RL 3rd, Beer B, et al. The cholinergic hypothesis of geriatric memory dysfunction. Science 1982;217(4558):408–14.
6. Adlimoghaddam A, Neuendorff M, Roy B, et al. A review of clinical treatment considerations of donepezil in severe Alzheimer's disease. CNS Neurosci Ther 2018; 24(10):876–88.
7. Xu H, Garcia-Ptacek S, Jönsson L, et al. Long-term effects of cholinesterase inhibitors on cognitive decline and mortality. Neurology 2021;96(17): e2220–30.
8. Attems Johannes, Jellinger Kurt. The overlap between vascular disease and Alzheimer's disease – lessons from pathology. BMC Med 2014;12:206.
9. Matsunaga S, Kishi T, Yasue I, et al. Cholinesterase inhibitors for Lewy Body disorders: a meta-analysis. Int J Neuropsychopharmacol 2015;19(2):pyv086.
10. Liu Mu-N, Chi-Ieong Lau, Ching-Po Lin. Precision medicine for frontotemporal dementia. Front Psychiatry 2019;10. https://doi.org/10.3389/fpsyt.2019.00075.
11. Russ TC, Morling JR. Cholinesterase inhibitors for mild cognitive impairment. Cochrane Database Syst Rev 2012;2012(9):CD009132.
12. Lee J-H, Jeong S-K, Kim BC, et al. Donepezil across the spectrum of Alzheimer's disease: dose optimization and clinical relevance. Acta Neurol Scand 2015; 131(5):259–67.
13. Pfizer Inc. Aricept (donepezil hydrochloride) [package insert]. U.S. Food and Drug Administration website. 2012. https://www.accessdata.fda.gov/

drugsatfda_docs/label/2012/020690s035,021720s008,022568s005lbl.pdf. [Accessed 31 August 2022].

14. Knopman DS. Donepezil 23 mg: an empty suit. Neurol Clin Pract 2012;2(4): 352–5.
15. Birks JS, Harvey RJ. Donepezil for dementia due to Alzheimer's disease. Cochrane Database Syst Rev 2018;6(6):CD001190.
16. Novartis. Exelon (rivastigmine tartrate) [package insert]. U.S. Food and Drug Administration website. 2018. https://www.accessdata.fda.gov/drugsatfda_docs/label/2018/020823s036,021025s024lbl.pdf. [Accessed 31 August 2022].
17. Birks JS, Grimley Evans J. Rivastigmine for Alzheimer's disease. Cochrane Database Syst Rev 2015;(4):CD001191.
18. Khoury R, Rajamanickam J, Grossberg GT. An update on the safety of current therapies for Alzheimer's disease: focus on rivastigmine. Ther Adv Drug Saf 2018;9(3):171–8.
19. Nordberg A, Ballard C, Bullock R, et al. A review of butyrylcholinesterase as a therapeutic target in the treatment of Alzheimer's disease. Prim Care Companion CNS Disord 2013;15(2). PCC.12r01412.
20. Ortho-McNeil Neurologics. Razadyne (galantamine hydrobromide) [package insert]. U.S. Food and Drug Administration website. 2015. https://www.accessdata.fda.gov/drugsatfda_docs/label/2015/021615s021lbl.pdf. [Accessed 31 August 2022].
21. Loy C, Schneider L. Galantamine for Alzheimer's disease and mild cognitive impairment. Cochrane Database Syst Rev 2006;2006(1):CD001747.
22. Kowal NM, Ahring PK, Liao VWY, et al. Galantamine is not a positive allosteric modulator of human α4β2 or α7 nicotinic acetylcholine receptors. Br J Pharmacol 2018;175(14):2911–25.
23. Bakker C, van der Aart J, Hart EP, et al. Safety, pharmacokinetics, and pharmacodynamics of Gln-1062, a prodrug of galantamine. Alzheimers Dement (N Y) 2020;6(1):e12093.
24. Forest Laboratories. Namenda (memantine HCl) [package insert]. U.S. Food and Drug Administration website. 2013. https://www.accessdata.fda.gov/drugsatfda_docs/label/2013/021487s010s012s014,021627s008lbl.pdf. [Accessed 31 August 2022].
25. McShane R, Westby MJ, Roberts E, et al. Memantine for dementia. Cochrane Database Syst Rev 2019;3(3):CD003154.
26. Dou KX, Tan MS, Tan CC, et al. Comparative safety and effectiveness of cholinesterase inhibitors and memantine for Alzheimer's disease: a network meta-analysis of 41 randomized controlled trials. Alzheimer's Res Ther 2018;10(1):126.
27. Hager K, Baseman AS, Nye JS, et al. Effects of galantamine in a 2-year, randomized, placebo-controlled study in Alzheimer's disease. Neuropsychiatr Dis Treat 2014;10:391–401.
28. Wilcock G, Möbius HJ, Stöffler A. MMM 500 group. A double-blind, placebo-controlled multicentre study of memantine in mild to moderate vascular dementia (MMM500). Int Clin Psychopharmacol 2002;17(6):297–305.
29. Orgogozo JM, Rigaud AS, Stöffler A, et al. Efficacy and safety of memantine in patients with mild to moderate vascular dementia: a randomized, placebo-controlled trial (MMM 300). Stroke 2002;33(7):1834–9.
30. Tan C-C, Yu J-T, Wang H-F, et al. Efficacy and safety of donepezil, galantamine, rivastigmine, and memantine for the treatment of Alzheimer's disease: a systematic review and meta-analysis. J Alzhemiers Dis 2014;41:615–31.

31. Hansen RA, Gartlehner G, Webb AP, et al. Efficacy and safety of donepezil, galantamine, and rivastigmine for the treatment of Alzheimer's disease: a systematic review and meta-analysis. Clin Interv Aging 2008;3(2):211–25.
32. Guo J, Wang Z, Liu R, et al. Memantine, donepezil, or combination therapy-What is the best therapy for Alzheimer's disease? A network meta-analysis. Brain Behav 2020;10(11):e01831.
33. Campbell NL, Perkins AJ, Gao S, et al. Adherence and tolerability of Alzheimer's disease medications: a Pragmatic randomized trial. J Am Geriatr Soc 2017;65(7): 1497–504.
34. Matsunaga S, Kishi T, Nomura I, et al. The efficacy and safety of memantine for the treatment of Alzheimer's disease. Expert Opin Drug Saf 2018;17(10):1053–61.
35. Massoud F, Desmarais JE, Gauthier S. Switching cholinesterase inhibitors in older adults with dementia. Int Psychogeriatr 2011;23(3):372–8.
36. Courtney C, Farrell D, Gray R, et al. AD2000 Collaborative Group. Long-term donepezil treatment in 565 patients with Alzheimer's disease (AD2000): randomised double-blind trial. Lancet 2004;363(9427):2105–15.
37. Howard R, McShane R, Lindesay J, et al. Nursing home placement in the Donepezil and Memantine in Moderate to Severe Alzheimer's Disease (DOMINO-AD) trial: secondary and post hoc analyses. Lancet Neurol 2015;14:1171–81.
38. Ismail Z, Black SE, Camicioli R, et al. Recommendations of the 5th Canadian Consensus Conference on the diagnosis and treatment of dementia. Alzheimer's Dement 2020;16:1182–95.
39. Ostrowitzki S, Lasser RA, Dorflinger E, et al, SCarlet RoAD Investigators. A phase III randomized trial of gantenerumab in prodromal Alzheimer's disease. Alzheimers Res Ther 2017;9(1):95.
40. Honig LS, Vellas B, Woodward M, et al. Trial of solanezumab for mild dementia due to Alzheimer's disease. N Engl J Med 2018;378(4):321–30.
41. Schneider L. A resurrection of aducanumab for Alzheimer's disease. Lancet Neurol 2020;19(2):111–2.
42. Prins ND, Scheltens P. Treating Alzheimer's disease with monoclonal antibodies: current status and outlook for the future. Alz Res Ther 2013;5:56.
43. Baker J, Schott JM. AD and its comorbidities: an obstacle to develop a clinically efficient treatment? Rev Neurol (Paris) 2022. https://doi.org/10.1016/j.neurol.2022.03.001. S0035-3787(22)00546-X.
44. Dyer O. Medicare's decision not to fund Aduhelm changes the landscape for US pharma industry. BMJ 2022;377. https://doi.org/10.1136/bmj.o996.
45. Decourt B, Boumelhem F, Pope ED 3rd, et al. Critical Appraisal of amyloid Lowering agents in AD. Curr Neurol Neurosci Rep 2021;21(8):39.
46. Battle CE, Abdul-Rahim AH, Shenkin SD, et al. Cholinesterase inhibitors for vascular dementia and other vascular cognitive impairments: a network meta-analysis. Cochrane Database Syst Rev 2021;2(2):CD013306.
47. Jin BR, Liu HY. Comparative efficacy and safety of cognitive enhancers for treating vascular cognitive impairment: systematic review and Bayesian network meta-analysis. Neural Regen Res 2019;14(5):805–16.
48. Smith EE, Barber P, Field TS, et al. Canadian Consensus Conference on diagnosis and treatment of dementia (CCCDTD)5: guidelines for management of vascular cognitive impairment. Alzheimer's Dementia (New York, N Y.) 2020; 6(1):e12056.
49. Ryan J, Storey E, Murray AM, et al, ASPREE Investigator Group. Randomized placebo-controlled trial of the effects of aspirin on dementia and cognitive decline. Neurology 2020;95(3):e320–31.

50. AD2000 Collaborative Group, Bentham P, Gray R, Sellwood E, et al. Aspirin in Alzheimer's disease (AD2000): a randomised open-label trial. Lancet Neurol 2008; 7(1):41–9.

51. Thoonsen H, Riichard E, Bentham P, et al. Aspirin in Alzheimer's disease: increased risk of intracerebral hemorrhage: cause for concern? Stroke 2010; 41(11):2690–2.

52. Meschia JF, Bushnell C, Boden-Albala B, et al. Guidelines for the primary prevention of stroke: a statement for healthcare professionals from the American Heart association/American stroke association. Stroke 2014;45:3754–832.

53. Sara Mondini, Ileana Madella, Andrea Zangrossi, et al. Cognitive reserve in dementia: Implications for cognitive training. Front Aging Neurosci 2016;8. https://doi.org/10.3389/fnagi.2016.00084.

54. Sanches C, Stengel C, Godard J, et al. Past, present, and future of non-invasive brain stimulation approaches to Treat cognitive impairment in neurodegenerative diseases: time for a Comprehensive Critical review. Front Aging Neurosci 2021; 12:578339.

55. Zelinski EM. Far transfer in cognitive training of older adults. Restorative Neurol Neurosci 2009;27(5):455–71.

56. Bahar-Fuchs A, Martyr A, Goh AMY, et al. Cognitive training for people with mild to moderate dementia. Cochrane Database Syst Rev 2019;(3):CD013069.

57. Hill NT, Mowszowski L, Naismith SL, et al. Computerized cognitive training in older adults with mild cognitive impairment or dementia: a systematic review and meta-analysis. Am J Psychiatry 2017;174(4):329–40.

58. Phan SV, Osae S, Morgan JC, et al. Neuropsychiatric symptoms in dementia: considerations for Pharmacotherapy in the USA. Drugs R D 2019;19(2):93–115.

59. Lyketsos CG, Lopez O, Jones B, et al. Prevalence of neuropsychiatric symptoms in dementia and mild cognitive impairment: Results from the cardiovascular health study. JAMA 2002;288(12):1475–83.

60. Ismail Z, McGirr A, Gill S, et al. Mild behavioral impairment and Subjective cognitive decline predict cognitive and functional decline. J Alzheimers Dis 2021;80(1): 459–69.

61. Wancata J, Windhaber J, Krautgartner M, et al. The consequences of non-cognitive symptoms of dementia in medical hospital departments. Int J Psychiatry Med 2003;33(3):257–71.

62. By the 2019 American Geriatrics Society Beers Criteria® Update Expert Panel. American Geriatrics society 2019 Updated AGS Beers Criteria® for Potentially Inappropriate medication Use in older adults. J Am Geriatr Soc 2019;67(4): 674–94.

63. Schneider LS, Dagerman KS, Insel P. Risk of death with atypical antipsychotic drug treatment for dementia: meta-analysis of randomized placebo-controlled trials. JAMA 2005;294(15):1934–43.

64. Cipriani G, Lucetti C, Nuti A, et al. Wandering and dementia. Psychogeriatrics 2014;14(2):135–42.

65. Neubauer NA, Azad-Khaneghah P, Miguel-Cruz A, et al. What do we know about strategies to manage dementia-related wandering? A scoping review. Alzheimers Demen 2018;10:615–28.

66. Montero-Odasso M, Verghese J, Beauchet O, et al. Gait and cognition: a complementary approach to understanding brain function and the risk of falling. J Am Geriatr Soc 2012;60(11):2127–36.

67. Zhang W, Low LF, Schwenk M, et al. Review of Gait, cognition, and fall risks with Implications for fall prevention in older adults with dementia. Dement Geriatr Cogn Disord 2019;48(1–2):17–29.

68. Racey M, Markle-Reid M, Fitzpatrick-Lewis D, et al. Fall prevention in community-dwelling adults with mild to moderate cognitive impairment: a systematic review and meta-analysis. BMC Geriatr 2021;21(1):689.

69. Morello RT, Soh SE, Behm K, et al. Multifactorial falls prevention programmes for older adults presenting to the emergency department with a fall: systematic review and meta-analysis. Inj Prev 2019;25(6):557–64.

70. Lord SR, Close JCT. New horizons in falls prevention. Age Ageing 2018;47(4): 492–8.

71. Lee L, Molnar F. Driving and dementia: efficient approach to driving safety concerns in family practice. Can Fam Physician 2017;63(1):27–31.

72. Breen DA, Breen DP, Moore JW, et al. Driving and dementia. BMJ 2007; 334(7608):1365–9.

73. Jacobs M, Hart EP, Roos RAC. Driving with a neurodegenerative disorder: an overview of the current literature. J Neurol 2017;264(8):1678–96.

74. Stamatelos P, Economou A, Stefanis L, et al. Driving and Alzheimer's dementia or mild cognitive impairment: a systematic review of the existing guidelines emphasizing on the neurologist's role. Neurol Sci 2021;42(12):4953–63.

75. Polzer ER, Nearing KA, Knoepke CE, et al. Firearm access and dementia: a qualitative study of reported behavioral disturbances and responses. J Am Geriatr Soc 2022;70(2):439–48.

76. Schwertner E, Zelic R, Secnik J, et al. Biting the Bullet: firearm ownership in persons with dementia. A Registry-based Observational study. J Alzheimers Dis 2021;81(1):179–88.

77. Pinholt EM, Mitchell JD, Butler JH, et al. Is there a gun in the home?" Assessing the risks of gun ownership in older adults. J Am Geriatr Soc 2014;62(6):1142–6.

78. Lee S, Kirk A, Kirk EA, et al. Factors associated with having a will, power of attorney, and advanced healthcare Directive in patients presenting to a Rural and Remote memory clinic. Can J Neurol Sci 2019;46(3):319–30.

79. Sellars M, Chung O, Nolte L, et al. Perspectives of people with dementia and carers on advance care planning and end-of-life care: a systematic review and thematic synthesis of qualitative studies. Palliat Med 2019;33(3):274–90.

80. Manthorpe J, Samsi K. Person-centered dementia care: current perspectives. Clin Interv Aging 2016;11:1733–40.

81. Wendrich-van Dael A, Bunn F, Lynch J, et al. Advance care planning for people living with dementia: an umbrella review of effectiveness and experiences. Int J Nurs Stud 2020;107:103576.

82. Cheng ST. Dementia caregiver Burden: a research update and Critical analysis. Curr Psychiatry Rep 2017;19(9):64.

83. Chien LY, Chu H, Guo JL, et al. Caregiver support groups in patients with dementia: a meta-analysis. Int J Geriatr Psychiatry 2011;26(10):1089–98.

84. Tretteteig S, Vatne S, Rokstad AM. The influence of day care centres designed for people with dementia on family caregivers - a qualitative study. BMC Geriatr 2017;17(1):5.

85. Swan K, Hopper M, Wenke R, et al. Speech-language pathologist interventions for Communication in moderate-severe dementia: a systematic review. Am J Speech Lang Pathol 2018;27(2):836–52.

86. Bennett S, Laver K, Voigt-Radloff S, et al. Occupational therapy for people with dementia and their family carers provided at home: a systematic review and meta-analysis. BMJ Open 2019;9(11):e026308.
87. Zhu XC, Yu Y, Wang HF, et al. Physiotherapy intervention in Alzheimer's disease: systematic review and meta-analysis. J Alzheimers Dis 2015;44(1): 163–74.

Brain Reserve, Resilience, and Cognitive Stimulation Across the Lifespan

How Do These Factors Influence Risk of Cognitive Impairment and the Dementias?

Farzaneh A. Sorond, MD, PhD*, Philip B. Gorelick, MD, MPH

KEYWORDS

- Cognitive resilience • Cognitive reserve • Brain reserve • Brain health

KEY POINTS

- A subset of individuals identified at autopsy as having a lesion burden that would be expected to have caused cognitive impairment during life, seem to have remained clinically unaffected.
- Understanding the mismatch between lesion burden and cognition could provide insights into key mechanisms for maintaining cognitive health in old age and potentially lead to novel therapeutic opportunities.
- On the basis of the existing data multidomain interventions targeting risk factors across sociodemographic, clinical, and environmental and lifestyle habits are likely to decrease the incidence of dementia.
- Patient and caregiver education is a critical first step toward implementing interventions that require behavioral and lifestyle changes.

INTRODUCTION

With increasing lifespan, the aging brain is exposed to the progressive and gradual accumulation of changes in structure and function; changes that are detrimental to successful aging and increase the risk of age-related cognitive decline and dementia. Yet, there is currently no substantial disease-modifying treatment of dementia. Identifying strategies that build, enhance, and preserve cognition and promote successful brain aging may provide opportunities for prevention. Indeed, there is increasing recognition of concepts related to brain reserve, cognitive reserve, maintenance,

Department of Neurology, Division of Stroke, Northwestern University, Feinberg School of Medicine, 625 North Michigan Avenue, 11th Floor, Chicago, IL 60611, USA
* Corresponding author.
E-mail address: fsorond@nm.org

Clin Geriatr Med 39 (2023) 151–160
https://doi.org/10.1016/j.cger.2022.08.003
0749-0690/23/© 2022 Elsevier Inc. All rights reserved.

and compensation and their contribution to resilience within the research community. However, as theoretical and difficult to measure entities, these concepts are not yielding significant scientific innovations. To probe the mechanistic underpinnings of resilience, reserve, maintenance, and compensation as potential therapeutic targets for maintaining good cognition despite dementia-related neuropathologic changes, we must first define them and be able to measure them. In this section, we (i) discuss proposed definitions and constructs that may be amenable to mechanistic studies, (ii) review the limited available empirical human data, and (iii) summarize recommendations for the practicing clinicians and geriatricians who provide care for older adults.

DEFINITIONS

Early observations by Grünthal (1927) and Gellerstedt (1933) had already shown that neuropathological changes such as plaques, neurofibrillary tangles, and granulovacuolar degeneration could be shown in the brains of cognitively normal old people studied postmortem. Yet, empirical support for the concept of individual resilience as an explanation for the observed mismatch between the burden of brain pathology and antemortem cognitive performance started emerging in the 1960s.[1] In the nearly 100 years since Grünthal's observations, there has been a significant expansion in publications and terminology coined to describe the observed clinical-neuropathological dissociated patterns in cognitive brain aging. Terms such as reserve, resilience, compensation, and maintenance attributable to the brain (structure) and/or cognition (function) are increasingly propagated in emerging literature. However, these terms vary across distinct and overlapping definitions and pose significant barriers to the harmonization and execution of mechanistic studies. For any meaningful progress in the field, the challenge of measuring resilience, reserve, and resistance and evaluating the validity of the specific indicators of these concepts must be addressed.

One suggested approach has been to differentiate brain reserve from the cognitive reserve in the same way that we would differentiate hardware and software in the context of a computer.[1] In this analogy, brain reserve is a physical trait and relates to anatomical attributes, whereas cognitive reserve reflects compensatory mechanisms based on innate intelligence and life experiences. However, these concepts and definitions are interdependent and in practice, difficult to be differentiated in humans. To address this limitation, researchers have turned to animal models to look for elements of brain structure and function that are common across species and have tried to extrapolate insights gained from these studies to humans. Data from animal studies have established that age-related memory decline is not a result of cell death. In fact, there are no age-related differences in the abundance of the primary cell types of the hippocampus, the brain structure central to the formation of new memories.[2,3] As a result, the focus has now turned to understanding if neuronal dysfunction and loss of processes such neuronal plasticity and connectivity may be the mechanisms responsible for age-related cognitive decline. Within this framework, preserved neuronal plasticity and connectivity would be substrates for age-related cognitive resilience and reserve. For example, one hypothesis may be that higher educational attainment results in denser and stronger neuronal networks that provide for higher functional stability when faced with age-related challenges and ensure that the individual is less susceptible to cognitive decline. However, to be able to test these hypotheses, we need translational strategies that more effectively bridge animal models with human aging research. Mathematical models to operationalize the theoretical concept of reserve and resilience may also provide an opportunity to further test such hypotheses. These models approach reserve as a latent variable that cannot be measured directly.[4] For example, it is possible that some yet-unknown factor influences educational attainment and the subsequent manifestation of reserve, and it is that unknown factor, rather than educational attainment, that makes an individual less susceptible to cognitive decline.

Another operational definition and quantification proposed by Montine and colleagues[5] offers a different path toward identifying strategies and mechanisms that preserve cognitive function and promote successful aging. In their model, they specifically define and build a construct around three concepts of *resistance, resilience,* and *reserve* in the context of cognitive brain aging. *Resilience* reflects preserved activity despite injury. They further extend this definition to distinguish *apparent* from *essential resilience*. In other words, one can *appear* to be resilient to existing pathology because of one's resistance (*essential resilience*) to comorbid pathologies. *Resistance* is reflective of defensive mechanisms in response to injury. These mechanisms may be *intrinsic* (biological) or *environmental* (behavioral; avoiding exposure for example). Finally, *reserve*, is defined as pre-morbid capacity (eg, synaptic density or educational attainment) to sustain activity despite some level of injury and is distinguished from *compensation*, which reflects a post-injury mechanism to sustain activity (eg, recruitment of additional resources).

The aforementioned concepts play an important role in a shift in our understanding of dementias (eg, Alzheimer's disease [AD]) from syndromal manifestations (symptoms and signs) to biological constructs.[6] Currently, research focus in relation to the diagnosis of AD emphasizes the use of biomarkers such as beta-amyloid deposition, pathologic tau, and neurodegeneration in a system referred to as the ATN classification.[6] Therefore, AD may be considered on a continuum of biomarker changes and in prodromal stages that may lead to cognitive impairment, and provide biological targets for interventions to avert the disease process from moving forward before it is too late. Simply put, *resistance* refers to the ability of the brain to avoid age-related neuropathological changes but maintain the preservation of brain integrity and function despite inherent risks (eg, advancing age, genetic predisposition); whereas *resilience* is the brain's ability to handle concurrent neuropathological changes, yet maintain the preservation of the brain and its function.[7]

Resilience

Resilience, as a universal property across many complex systems, including the brain, refers to the ability of that system to maintain its functionality in the face of internal or external challenges. Data from *The 90+ Study*[8] provide preliminary support for the model and definitions proposed by Montine and colleagues[5] More specifically, these data show that neuropathological resilience to the non-AD pathologies (*essential resilience*) may result in cognitive resilience (*apparent* resilience) as AD pathology develops. Among 185 individuals from *The 90+ Study* with postmortem data, those with minimal cerebrovascular and other non-AD pathologies seemed to be more cognitively resilient to AD neuropathology.[8]

Reserve

Despite the wealth of scientific knowledge afforded by reductionism, the concepts, and pathways that explain resilience and reserve, transcend individual cellular components and their functions. To understand the network of interactions that contribute to the structure and function of a living cell, an organ, or an organism, we must embrace a systems approach. In fact, neuronal network connectivity may be a game-changer for successful brain aging.[9] Complex structural and functional connectivity is a distinctive feature of the human brain. On the basis of the graph theory, the brain can be modeled as a multifaceted operational network composed of nodes (neurons or brain regions, gray matter) linked by edges (synapses), and large-scale white matter tracts.[10] Strength of connectivity of portions of the network may vary and determine the relative importance of that component of the network to function. Previous studies have shown that in patients with dementia, there are specific neuronal networks that are frequently disrupted (eg, default mode network in AD that functions to monitor quiescent brain activity).[11] Furthermore, it has been shown that subtle changes in white matter microstructure are related to impaired global and local network efficiency and decreased network strength.[12] Similarly, for those with mild cognitive impairment (MCI), stronger functional network connectivity is associated with a slower pace of cognitive decline and progression to dementia.[13]

We have recently shown that greater connectivity of a left executive functional connectivity network (ECN) to the bilateral anterior gyrus rectus, right posterior orbitofrontal cortex, and nucleus accumbens was associated with better executive control performance on the Stroop executive task in midlife individuals with evidence of microvascular white matter injury. Our findings suggest that increased connectivity of the left ECN to regions involved in reward processing may compensate for the deleterious effects of microvascular lesions on executive function.[14] However, whether this connectivity is an example of *reserve* or *compensation*, as defined by Montine and colleagues[5] is not clear. Moreover, it is not known if the increased connectivity was a developmental feature in these individuals or an acquired feature that occurred in response to increasing white matter microvascular injury.

Resistance

Finally, we consider the construct of *resistance*, specifically *intrinsic resistance*. Why do only some individuals with hypertension have an intracranial hemorrhage, lacunar stroke, or white matter disease, and others do not? Similarly, why are some individuals resistant to the deleterious effects of neuropathology and able to maintain a successful cognitive aging trajectory? What are the endogenous and exogenous factors and their interactions that promote biological resistance in these individuals? For example, among 367 available autopsies from *The 90+ Study*, the brain belonging to the one participant who maintained normal cognition despite intermediate-high levels of three dementia-related neuropathologic changes (AD neuropathologic change [Thal phase 5, Braak NFT stage IV, CERAD score 3], Lewy bodies and neurites in the olfactory bulb, brainstem and limbic areas [Braak PD stage 4], TDP-43 inclusions in the amygdala and hippocampus [LATE stage 2]), only had one microvascular lesion in the putamen.[15] Interestingly, this person also had atrial fibrillation, congestive heart failure, and hypertension; yet somehow was resistant to microvascular pathology and cerebral ischemic lesions. Although healthy aging choices clearly lower the burden of vascular risk factors and reduce a person's dementia risk in old age, resistance to cerebrovascular pathology in the presence of vascular risk factors is an entirely different concept; one that remains unexplored.

STRATEGIES FOR SUCCESSFUL COGNITIVE AGING (WHAT, WHEN, AND WHOM)

Emerging evidence suggests that strategies to build, enhance, and preserve cognition and promote successful brain aging are dynamic constructs that span across the lifecourse and involve processes that begin early in life.[16] In data from 1697 dementia-free older participants from the Rush Memory and Aging Project, higher education, more cognitive activities during early, mid- and late-life, as well as late-life social activities were associated with a slower decline in cognitive function despite presence of significant neurodegenerative and ischemic pathologies.[17] Similarly, in the Uppsala Birth Cohort Multigenerational Study,[18] with an average of 21 years of follow-up in 7,574 participants, dementia risk was lower among individuals with higher grades in primary school. Another variable associated with reduced risk of dementia was high occupational complexity with data, but not with people or things. In fact, the lowest risk of dementia was found in individuals who leveraged higher school grades into complex occupational roles in adulthood. One possible hypothesis suggested by these data may be that the protection afforded by education is only realized when it is supplemented across the life span by continued cognitively demanding activities.[19] In other words, although early life factors are critical, successful cognitive aging requires that one continues to build on the structure and function of the brain across all life stages. Therefore, by incorporating activities that preserve brain health and avoiding those that are deleterious, we may be able to alter the trajectory of cognitive change across the prolonged preclinical phase of neurodegenerative disorders. Studies show that in addition to mental and physical stimulation early in and throughout the life course, nutrition, access to health care, psychosocial factors, and accumulation of vascular risk factors are additional exposures that modify genetic predisposition to cognitive outcomes and alter the course of brain health. Data that support benefits of diet, physical activity, and cognitive stimulation for successful cognitive aging are summarized below. However, our knowledge gap on the when and which approach to implement across different populations is a significant limitation to meaningfully enhancing brain health and cognitive function across the life span. Of importance are studies that have shown that in persons genetically predisposed to cognitively impairing disorders, favorable lifestyle and vascular risk factor profiles may attenuate the risk of cognitive impairment and dementia later in life.[20,21]

Diet. Adherence to a Mediterranean dietary pattern is associated with a lower risk of cognitive decline, and development of MCI and dementia. Late-life healthful diet may modulate cognitive performance independently of the early acquired cognitive reserve as assessed by the intelligence quotient. For example, in 120 Scottish individuals born in 1936 with cognitive measures at ages 64 and 68 years, those with higher levels of total omega-3 fatty acids at age 64 had better cognition at both time points regardless of their gender, early life IQ, or ApoE4 status.[22] The recent Spanish RCT PREDIMED also showed that a Mediterranean-style diet can prevent cardiovascular disease in high-risk asymptomatic adults aged 55–80 years and preserve cognitive function over 6.5 years of follow-up.[23] Similarly, a low glycemic index and low-fat diet were also associated with improved visual memory in those with MCI.[24]

Physical activity. The beneficial effects of exercise on preserving brain health are also well established and it is possible that the benefits stem from the prevention of chronic diseases associated with dementia.[25] Experimental models show exercise mediated upregulation of brain-derived neurotrophic factor and insulin-like growth factor 1, which are known to benefit angiogenesis and neuronal plasticity.[26] However, across a birth cohort born in 1972–1973 in New Zealand, higher cognitive performance during childhood was also associated with higher cardiorespiratory fitness 25 years later,[27] suggesting that the relationship between physical and cognitive fitness may be bidirectional.

Studies show that when older adults were able to significantly increase their cardiorespiratory fitness (assessed by VO_2 max), they often also achieved enhanced cognitive performance.[28,29] Even among frail individuals physical activity seems to be a promising intervention to prevent age-related cognitive decline and neurodegenration.[26,30] A 6-month program of aerobic exercise was associated with improved executive function in older adults with MCI,[29] and a 1-year program in obese older adults was associated with improved global cognitive function and executive functions.[31] These data suggest that even among older adults with MCI and obesity, exercise can prevent or slow cognitive decline.

Cognitive stimulation. Social and intellectual leisure activities also seem to have a beneficial impact on cognitive trajectories. Lifetime involvement in challenging life situations and intellectual leisure activities, whether professional or personal, is associated with cognitive reserve and slows neurodegeneration.[32] Data from the French Three-City study show that stimulating leisure activities, rather than passive leisure activities such as watching TV or knitting, specifically contributed to cognitive reserve.[33] Thus, the promotion of cognitively stimulating activities in older community-dwelling adults shows promise as a prevention strategy that could delay dementia onset. Data from the ACTIVE single-blind RCT show that the beneficial impact of cognitively stimulating activities can last up to 5 years following training.[34] Findings from various cognitive intervention programs also show a significant improvement in memory, quality of life, and mood, even among individuals with MCI.[35,36]

Other factors. Systemic reviews and meta-analyses verify significant associations between levels of resistance and resilience with the risk of progression of AD or dementia.[37] Furthermore, MCI, and intermediary clinical points in the pathway to AD or dementia, may revert to normal cognition when there are higher levels of cognitive reserve (eg, educational attainment, academic performance in high school, and written language skills in relation to idea density and grammatical complexity).[38] Even in the presence of brain pathologies predisposing to cognitive impairment (eg, substantial AD neuropathology or gross brain infarction), high cognitive reserve indicators may be associated with relative preservation of global cognitive function, episodic memory, and working memory.[17] Novel potential mediators of this effect include the X chromosome and cortical resilience proteins, respectively.[39,40] Whether vascular brain injury and the associated cognitive impairment are attenuated by the cognitive reserve, remains unkown.[41]

Multidomain Approach

Despite the reality that implementing beneficial lifestyle habits is difficult even though they pose no impediment to safety and may result in better vascular health, addressing these factors (diet, social engagement, cognitive stimulation, physical, exercise) remains the most reasonable target for promoting successful cognitive aging. However, because late-life dementia is a multi-factorial disorder, interventions targeting several risk factors simultaneously may be necessary to achieve the optimal preventive effect. Results from the FINGER intervention show that a multidomain approach was associated with overall cognition (primary outcome), executive function, and cognitive speed, as well as improved body mass index, food habits, and physical activity (secondary outcomes).

When Should Lifestyle Interventions be Carried out?

Prevention can be primordial or primary. Primordial prevention is about reducing disease incidence by preventing the occurrence of specific risk factors through promotion and maintenance of good health. Primary prevention is about targeting early prevention of disease by identification of clinical or biological markers that could lead to early detection and treatment of at-risk individuals. However, the optimal window for preventive interventions targeted at dementia is not known. Should the focus be on healthy individuals for primordial or primary prevention, or will those with mild cognitive symptoms also benefit from secondary prevention? Data summarized thus far suggest that both primordial, primary, and secondary prevention efforts are beneficial for promoting successful cognitive aging. Data also suggest that we should focus on preventing the biological processes underlying cognitive impairment rather than waiting until there are syndromic manifestations such as memory loss or other cognitive features that are clinical expressions of dementia. The balance between optimal timing of the intervention, the duration of intervention, and the incidence of the cognitive outcomes is not known and is difficult to ascertain. Earlier and longer interventions could result in greater treatment effects, but RCTs assessing their impact are sensitive to attrition. The average follow-up in prevention studies on vascular interventions with dementia as a secondary outcome has been 3 to 5 years though some non-dementia prevention RCTs have had follow-up of up to 10 years.[42]

Therefore, considering the existing knowledge gaps about the specific intervention that results in successful cognitive aging, it is reasonable to pursue a broad multiprong epidemiological approach to target risk factors across sociodemographic, clinical, and environmental, and lifestyle habits that will likely reduce the incidence of dementia and cognitive impairment. The goal of any multidomain approach should be to prevent injury (promote intrinsic and environmental *resistance*) and preserve cognition (build *reserve*, be *resilient* to injury through repair and compensation) across the life course. However, one must remain cognizant of the limitations inherent to the principles of interventional epidemiology and the existing construct of preventive strategies. We are limited to study what is available and gather data on what is measurable. Autonomy, purpose, social participation, and engagement are specific examples of variables that likely impact multimodal interventions but are too complex to measure and modify.

SUMMARY

Preserving cognitive function is essential for successful aging and a major challenge confronting our aging population. As reviewed in this article, cognitive health depends on the interaction of multiple determinants throughout the life span. Lifestyle factors can positively or negatively moderate dementia risk via neuropathological changes. Estimates suggest that up to 3 million dementia cases worldwide could be prevented if it was possible to reduce known risk factors by 25%.[43] Clearly, there is a need to implement public health policies that prevent cognitive decline and dementia, but educating our patients and communities may be the most important first step. In a recent survey of 3,130 individuals over the age of 40 conducted in the United Kingdom, most respondents believed that genes and lifestyle factors had an equal contribution to changes in cognitive skills and men, more than women believed that cognitive skills were predominantly influenced by our genes and were less modifiable across the life course.[44] This belief poses a significant impediment to an individual engaging in activities and behaviors that could positively impact successful cognitive aging. Primary care physicians are best poised to educate and engage at-risk individuals as early as possible and empowering them to take personal ownership of developing habits and behaviors that optimize successful cognitive aging throughout their life course.

CLINICS CARE POINTS

- In the absence of effective interventions to treat cognitive impairment and dementia, clinical focus must fall on the prevention and promotion of successful cognitive aging
- Existing data show that lifestyle factors can alter the trajectory of cognitive aging

- Implementation of multidomain interventions that target risk factors across sociodemographic, clinical, and environmental and lifestyle habits hold promise for reducing the incidence of dementia
- Patient and caregiver education on the importance of lifestyle factors is a critical first step toward successful implementation of multidomain interventions that require behavioral and lifestyle changes.

REFERENCES

1. Blessed G, Tomlinson BE, Roth M. The association between quantitative measures of dementia and of senile change in the cerebral grey matter of elderly subjects. Br J Psychiatry 1968;114(512):797–811.
2. Keuker JI, Luiten PG, Fuchs E. Preservation of hippocampal neuron numbers in aged rhesus monkeys. Neurobiol Aging 2003;24(1):157–65.
3. Rapp PR, Gallagher M. Preserved neuron number in the hippocampus of aged rats with spatial learning deficits. Proc Natl Acad Sci U S A 1996;93(18):9926–30.
4. Jones RN, Manly J, Glymour MM, et al. Conceptual and measurement challenges in research on cognitive reserve. J Int Neuropsychol Soc 2011;17(4):593–601.
5. Montine TJ, Cholerton BA, Corrada MM, et al. Concepts for brain aging: resistance, resilience, reserve, and compensation. Alzheimers Res Ther 2019; 11(1):22.
6. Jack CR Jr, Bennett DA, Blennow K, et al. NIA-AA Research Framework: toward a biological definition of Alzheimer's disease. Alzheimers Dement 2018;14(4): 535–62.
7. Poggesi A. Resilience and resistance in aging and alzheimer disease: another step to fill the gap between clinicians and researchers. Neurology 2021;97(10): 465–6.
8. Kawas CH, Kim RC, Sonnen JA, et al. Multiple pathologies are common and related to dementia in the oldest-old: the 90+ Study. Neurology 2015;85(6): 535–42.
9. Gao J, Barzel B, Barabasi AL. Universal resilience patterns in complex networks. Nature 2016;530(7590):307–12.
10. Iturria-Medina Y, Sotero RC, Canales-Rodriguez EJ, et al. Studying the human brain anatomical network via diffusion-weighted MRI and Graph Theory. Neuroimage 2008;40(3):1064–76.
11. Pievani M, de Haan W, Wu T, et al. Functional network disruption in the degenerative dementias. Lancet Neurol 2011;10(9):829–43.
12. Li S, Wang B, Xu P, et al. Increased global and local efficiency of human brain anatomical networks detected with FLAIR-DTI compared to non-FLAIR-DTI. PLoS One 2013;8(8):e71229.
13. Petrella JR, Sheldon FC, Prince SE, et al. Default mode network connectivity in stable vs progressive mild cognitive impairment. Neurology 2011;76(6):511–7.
14. Jenkins LM, Kogan A, Malinab M, et al. Blood pressure, executive function, and network connectivity in middle-aged adults at risk of dementia in late life. Proc Natl Acad Sci U S A 2021;118:37.
15. Melikyan ZA, Corrada MM, Leiby AM, et al. Cognitive resilience to three dementia-related neuropathologies in an oldest-old man: a case report from the 90+ Study. Neurobiol Aging 2022;116:12–5.
16. Lathrop DL, Griebel M, Horner J. Dysphagia in tetanus: evaluation and outcome. Dysphagia 1989;4(3):173–5.

17. Li X, Song R, Qi X, et al. Influence of cognitive reserve on cognitive trajectories: role of brain pathologies. Neurology 2021;97(17):e1695–706.
18. Dekhtyar S, Wang HX, Scott K, et al. A life-course study of cognitive reserve in dementia–from childhood to old age. Am J Geriatr Psychiatry 2015;23(9):885–96.
19. Orrell M, Sahakian B. Education and dementia. BMJ 1995;310(6985):951–2.
20. Dekhtyar S, Marseglia A, Xu W, et al. Genetic risk of dementia mitigated by cognitive reserve: a cohort study. Ann Neurol 2019;86(1):68–78.
21. Lourida I, Hannon E, Littlejohns TJ, et al. Association of lifestyle and genetic risk with incidence of dementia. JAMA 2019;322(5):430–7.
22. Whalley LJ, Deary IJ, Starr JM, et al. n-3 Fatty acid erythrocyte membrane content, APOE varepsilon4, and cognitive variation: an observational follow-up study in late adulthood. Am J Clin Nutr 2008;87(2):449–54.
23. Martinez-Lapiscina EH, Clavero P, Toledo E, et al. Mediterranean diet improves cognition: the PREDIMED-NAVARRA randomised trial. J Neurol Neurosurg Psychiatr 2013;84(12):1318–25.
24. Bayer-Carter JL, Green PS, Montine TJ, et al. Diet intervention and cerebrospinal fluid biomarkers in amnestic mild cognitive impairment. Arch Neurol 2011;68(6): 743–52.
25. Larson EB, Wang L, Bowen JD, et al. Exercise is associated with reduced risk for incident dementia among persons 65 years of age and older. Ann Intern Med 2006;144(2):73–81.
26. Bherer L, Frickson KI, Liu-Ambrose T. A review of the effects of physical activity and exercise on cognitive and brain functions in older adults. J Aging Res 2013; 2013:657508.
27. Belsky DW, Caspi A, Israel S, et al. Cardiorespiratory fitness and cognitive function in midlife: neuroprotection or neuroselection? Ann Neurol 2015;77(4):607–17.
28. Teychenne M, Ball K, Salmon J. Promoting physical activity and reducing sedentary behavior in disadvantaged neighborhoods: a qualitative study of what women want. PLoS One 2012;7(11):e49583.
29. Lautenschlager NT, Cox KL, Flicker L, et al. Effect of physical activity on cognitive function in older adults at risk for Alzheimer disease: a randomized trial. JAMA 2008;300(9):1027–37.
30. Bherer L, Erickson KI, Liu-Ambrose T. Physical exercise and brain functions in older adults. J Aging Res 2013;2013:197326.
31. Napoli N, Shah K, Waters DL, et al. Effect of weight loss, exercise, or both on cognition and quality of life in obese older adults. Am J Clin Nutr 2014;100(1): 189–98.
32. Scarmeas N, Stern Y. Cognitive reserve and lifestyle. J Clin Exp Neuropsychol 2003;25(5):625–33.
33. Akbaraly TN, Portet F, Fustinoni S, et al. Leisure activities and the risk of dementia in the elderly: results from the Three-City Study. Neurology 2009;73(11):854–61.
34. Willis SL, Tennstedt SL, Marsiske M, et al. Long-term effects of cognitive training on everyday functional outcomes in older adults. JAMA 2006;296(23):2805–14.
35. Mowszowski L, Batchelor J, Naismith SL. Early intervention for cognitive decline: can cognitive training be used as a selective prevention technique? Int Psychogeriatr 2010;22(4):537–48.
36. Jean L, Bergeron ME, Thivierge S, et al. Cognitive intervention programs for individuals with mild cognitive impairment: systematic review of the literature. Am J Geriatr Psychiatry 2010;18(4):281–96.

37. Bocancea DI, van Loenhoud AC, Groot C, et al. Measuring resilience and resistance in aging and alzheimer disease using residual methods: a systematic review and meta-analysis. Neurology 2021;97(10):474–88.

38. Iraniparast M, Shi Y, Wu Y, et al. Cognitive reserve and mild cognitive impairment: predictors and rates of reversion to intact cognition vs progression to dementia. Neurology 2022;98(11):e1114–23.

39. Davis EJ, Solsberg CW, White CC, et al. Sex-specific association of the X chromosome with cognitive change and tau pathology in aging and alzheimer disease. JAMA Neurol 2021;78(10):1249–54.

40. Zammit AR, Yu L, Petyuk V, et al. Cortical proteins and individual differences in cognitive resilience in older adults. Neurology 2022;98(13):e1304–14.

41. Durrani R, Friedrich MG, Schulze KM, et al. Effect of cognitive reserve on the association of vascular brain injury with cognition: analysis of the PURE and CAHHM studies. Neurology 2021;97(17):e1707–16.

42. Whiteley WN, Anand S, Bangdiwala SI, et al. Are large simple trials for dementia prevention possible? Age Ageing 2020;49(2):154–60.

43. Barnes DE, Yaffe K. The projected effect of risk factor reduction on Alzheimer's disease prevalence. Lancet Neurol 2011;10(9):819–28.

44. Niechcial MA, Vaportzis E, Gow AJ. Genes versus lifestyles: exploring beliefs about the determinants of cognitive ageing. Front Psychol 2022;13:838323.

Beyond Memory and Other Cognitive Dysfunction: Neurobehavioral and Psychiatric Disorders

Diagnostic and Management Strategies for Common Neurobehavioral and Psychiatric Disturbances Among Patients with Cognitive Impairment and the Dementias

Akashleena Mallick, MD, Alessandro Biffi, MD*

KEYWORDS

- Dementia • Cognitive impairment • Behavioral neurology • Neuropsychiatry
- Psychopharmacology

KEY POINTS

- Prompt diagnosis of behavioral and neuropsychiatric disorders in dementia care requires collaborative efforts including providers, patients, and caregivers.
- Health care providers should familiarize themselves with diagnostic tools targeting behavioral and neuropsychiatric symptoms, to facilitate diagnosis and guide management.
- Non-pharmacological interventions should be considered the first-line for the treatment of most behavioral and neuropsychiatric disorders, especially in elderly individuals.
- Judicious use of medications under the guidance of an expert practitioner is warranted to address symptoms severely impacting patients' safety and quality of life.

INTRODUCTION

Behavioral and neuropsychiatric symptoms (primarily in the form of anxiety, depression, psychosis, agitation, and aggression) are highly prevalent among individuals diagnosed with cognitive impairment or dementia. In a systematic review published in 2015, up to 90% of community-dwelling individuals diagnosed with dementia displayed evidence of one or more behavioral or neuropsychiatric symptoms (**Table 1**).[1] These conditions are associated with earlier functional decline and increased caregiver burden.[2] Prompt

The authors have nothing to disclose.
Department of Neurology, Massachusetts General Hospital and Harvard Medical School, Henry and Allison McCance Center for Brain Health, 100 Cambridge Street, Room 2054, Boston, MA 02144, USA
* Corresponding author.
E-mail address: abiffi@mgh.harvard.edu

Clin Geriatr Med 39 (2023) 161–175
https://doi.org/10.1016/j.cger.2022.08.004
0749-0690/23/© 2022 Elsevier Inc. All rights reserved.

Table 1		
Prevalence of behavioral and neuropsychiatric disturbances among patients with dementia		
Disorder	Point Prevalence	Cumulative Prevalence
Anxiety	18%–24%	43%–66%
Agitation/aggression	6%–26%	40%–74%
Apathy	23%–40%	43%–63%
Depression	10%–42%	20%–78%
Hallucinations	0%–43%	32%–70%
Delusions/psychosis	5%–61%	34%–80%
Sleep disturbances	9%–18%	25%–30%

Data from Borsje P, Wetzels RB, Lucassen PL, Pot AM, Koopmans RT. The course of neuropsychiatric symptoms in community-dwelling patients with dementia: a systematic review. International psychogeriatrics / IPA. 2015;27(3):385-405. Epub 2014/11/19. https://doi.org/10.1017/s1041610214002282. PubMed PMID: 25403309.

diagnosis and effective management of these conditions are therefore central to optimal patient and caregiver outcomes. This article provides guidance on the diagnostic approach to and management of common behavioral and neuropsychiatric disorders frequently affecting individuals diagnosed with cognitive impairment (up to an including dementia). In addition to general diagnostic and management strategies, we will discuss specific approaches to depression, anxiety, apathy, and psychosis in patients with cognitive impairment and dementia.

GENERAL DIAGNOSTIC APPROACH

In most instances, behavioral and neuropsychiatric symptoms are first noticed by caregivers in a patient already diagnosed with cognitive impairment or dementia.[3] In other instances (especially for individuals with milder forms of cognitive impairment), signs and symptoms are directly reported by patients.[1] It is therefore imperative to ensure patients and caregivers are familiar with common manifestations of behavioral and neuropsychiatric disorders (**Table 2**). Health care providers should specifically educate caregivers in using consistent, descriptive language when reporting patients' symptoms and behavior, to facilitate diagnosis and monitoring. A clear, succinct description of behaviors observed (eg, "repeatedly ignoring requests to perform tasks, associated with scoffing") is preferable to non-specific terms (eg, "irritable"). Likewise, caregivers should be consistently asked to clarify the consequences associated with active behavioral and neuropsychiatric symptoms (eg, "unable to participate in household chores"). Providers should also elicit information on frequency (eg, daily vs weekly) and timing of symptoms (time of day, and association with sleep, food, medication use, physical activity), as well as associated triggers and precipitating factors. These individual-specific details can be invaluable in devising specific management strategies, based on measurable treatment goals (eg, reduction in the frequency of disruptive anxiety symptoms from daily to weekly or less).

In addition to direct interviews to elicit the manifestations listed above, health care providers can use a variety of questionnaires to quantitatively assess behavioral and neuropsychiatric disorders complicating dementia. Because of cognitive impairment and behavioral or neuropsychiatric symptoms (eg, lack of engagement due to severe depression) formal psychometric testing is often unfeasible. We therefore recommend focusing on the administration of a standardized evaluation instrument for reliable informants, with the Neuro-Psychiatry Inventory (NPI) representing our preferred choice.[3] When feasible,

Table 2	
Common manifestations of behavioral and neuropsychiatric disorders among patients with dementia	
Disorder	**Manifestations**
Anxiety	Breathlessness, excessive worry, excessive fear of something bad happening, and excessive concerns about separation from a caregiver
Agitation/aggression	Excessive pacing, restlessness, repetitive movements, hitting/kicking, and screaming
Apathy	Decreased interest in participating in activities, decreased motivation, decreased energy level, and increased sleeping
Depression	Sadness, tearfulness, thought rumination, excessive self-deprecation, early morning awakenings, and mood-congruent delusions
Hallucinations	Hearing, seeing, or otherwise sensing inanimate things or individuals that are not real
Delusions/psychosis	False belief of someone trying to harm or steal from patient
Sleep disturbances	Repeated night-time awakenings, early morning awakenings, and excessive daytime napping

standardized neuropsychological tools can also be administered to patients to diagnose behavioral and neuropsychiatric disorders, to (1) confirm diagnostic impressions; (2) help guide the creation of a treatment plan for them. Selection of tests should be based primarily on practitioners' prior expertise and clinical setting.

Evaluation of behavioral and neuropsychiatric symptoms in patients with cognitive impairment should also always include an evaluation for potential superimposed delirium.[4] Delirium represents a very common occurrence in patients with dementia, and its manifestations (agitation, aggression, hallucinations) can closely mimic other neuropsychiatric conditions. A variety of tools are available for delirium screening, with the Confusion Assessment Method (CAM) being the most commonly implemented in clinical practice.[5] Finally, upon formulating a diagnosis of one or more behavioral or neuropsychiatric disorders, health care providers should complete a thorough evaluation (by history and examination) of factors that may affect underlying risk, onset, and clinical course(**Table 3**). These factors are critical in formulating a management approach, as well as in communicating prognosis and treatment plans to both patients and caregivers.

GENERAL MANAGEMENT STRATEGIES

Management of behavioral and neuropsychiatric symptoms is best approached using collaborative strategies involving patients, caregivers, and health care providers. Because symptoms are usually dynamically changing over time, health care providers are encouraged to use a multi-step approach to care while setting up specific measurable goals. Patient and caregivers can then be tasked with symptom monitoring (either informally, or using recording tools) to monitor progress.[6] We recommend that health care providers work closely with patients and caregivers on a dementia care plan that incorporates: (1) initial setting and evaluation of treatment goals, (2) longitudinal follow-up for re-evaluation, and (3) updated intervention measures. Individuals' personal values, financial resources, social circumstances, and local resources of the patients are also crucial in tailoring intervention measures.

Table 3
Factors contributing to onset and course of behavioral and neuropsychiatric disorders in patients with cognitive impairment and dementia

Protective	Predisposing	Precipitating	Perpetuating
Familiar individuals	Challenging environment	Pain level	Inadequate Patient–caregiver Communication
Familiar environment	Hearing impairment	Hunger	Delayed diagnosis
Caregiver expertise	Vision impairment	Thirst	Inadequate treatment
Caregiver support	Caregiver stress	Medication changes	No pre-formulated dementia care plan
Pre-formulated dementia care plan	Dementia severity	Temperature extremes	Limited support for caregiver
	Comorbid psychiatric conditions	Sleep disruption	

From a general standpoint, management strategies aimed at addressing behavioral and neuropsychiatric symptoms can be classified as either pharmacological or non-pharmacological. In most circumstances, consideration of safety and overall efficacy have prompted guidelines to recommend the implementation of non-pharmacological management strategies first. Such treatment modalities (**Table 4**) include psychological therapies, psychosocial interventions, and environmental modifications. In two studies conducted in high-income countries across different care settings, various non-pharmacological intervention methods resulted in a clinically meaningful reduction in neuropsychiatric symptoms in patients with dementia.[7,8] In addition, all caregivers should receive training aimed at implementing basic, easy-to-deploy non-pharmacological interventions.[9]

Pharmacological interventions (especially use of antipsychotic drugs) should only be considered when absolutely necessary. Typical indications include: (1) patient in severe distress due to behavioral or neuropsychiatric symptoms, (2) patient is at risk of self-harm, either because of behavioral impairment or inability to self-care, and (3) patient represents a potential threat to people surrounding them. Overall, use of medications to treat behavioral and neuropsychiatric symptoms in patients with dementia requires a deliberate effort to consistently discuss treatment goals with patients and caregivers, and establish timelines for review of symptoms and potential side effects. Use of antipsychotic drugs, in particular, has been associated with potential harms in dementia patients, including increased risk of stroke, falls and traumatic fractures, and death.[10–13] As a result, their use is reducing or stabilizing in countries such as Canada, the United States, and the United Kingdom.[14–16] Deprescribing antipsychotic agents should always be considered based on symptoms' evolution. There are no established guidelines to deprescribing, but slowly tapering of antipsychotics (25% to 50% dose reduction every two weeks until discontinuation) under the guidance of an expert clinician is generally appropriate.

DISORDER-SPECIFIC DIAGNOSTIC AND TREATMENT CONSIDERATIONS
Anxiety

Definition and pathogenesis. Anxiety is defined as a subjective perception of threat or danger associated with anticipated events, induced internally or externally, that can interfere with normally daily activities. These persistent and excessive feelings

Table 4
Non-pharmacological treatment options for behavioral and neuropsychiatric disorders in patients with cognitive impairment and dementia

Intervention	Brief Description
Music therapy	Therapy focused on auditory feedback to achieve changes in emotional states
Animal therapy	Therapy involving exposure to trained animals to achieve changes in emotional states
Cognitive stimulation	Structured sessions (conducted at least weekly) aimed at promoting performance in specific cognitive tasks (eg, memory recall)
Occupational therapy	Structured sessions (conducted at least weekly) aimed at promoting functional independence in tasks critical for patient's safety, independence, and sense of self-worth
Physical exercise	Any combination of aerobic, endurance, and balance training physical activity
Massage and touch therapy	Sensory feedback-based therapies, including massage, acupuncture, and therapeutic touch
Reminiscence therapy	Therapy leveraging patient's positive memories to achieve relaxation and promote positive adoptive responses
Psychotherapy	Group of treatment modalities (including cognitive-behavioral therapy, dialectic therapy, individual and group counseling) aimed at achieving positive changes in emotional states
Social interactions	Active social interactions with others, outside the boundaries of employment or provision of care (eg, volunteering)
Environmental modifications	Changes in patient's living situation (physical and psychosocial) targeting factors influencing behavioral and cognitive symptoms

of worry, fear, panic, and restlessness occur frequently for at least six months. In contrast, occasional instances of nervousness or stress are considered normal, and do not disable daily functioning. Anxiety-spectrum disorders are the most common mental health condition, impacting nearly 30% of adults.[17] From a neurochemistry standpoint, the most critical mediators of anxiety in the central nervous system are norepinephrine, serotonin, dopamine, and gamma-aminobutyric acid (GABA). The autonomic nervous system, particularly the sympathetic nervous system, modulates most of the symptoms. From a connectivity standpoint, the amygdala and limbic system structures and their connections to the prefrontal cortex regions are central to pathogenesis.[18–20] Although anxiety disorders are known to be highly heritable, only a handful of genetic loci have to date been identified as associated with disease risk.[20]

Diagnosis. formal diagnosis of anxiety in the setting of cognitive impairment or dementia uses the same diagnostic categories applicable to the general population, as laid out in the Diagnostic and Statistical Manual of Mental Disorders (DSM-5).[21] Health care providers can also use other structured interview tools, including the WHO's Composite International Diagnostic Interview, and the Mini-International Neuropsychiatric Interview.[22] Alternatively, assessment can leverage several standardized self-administered or informant questionnaires including the Rating Anxiety In Dementia (RAID) scale, the Generalized Anxiety Disorder 7-Items (GAD-7) scale, or the Overall Anxiety Severity and Impairment Scale (OASIS) for an initial assessment.[23] More in-depth psychometric testing can be considered, under the guidance of an expert neuropsychologist, to evaluate for situation-specific anxiety and phobias that would otherwise escape characterization. At present, no specific biomarkers (serological, in cerebrospinal fluid [CSF], or neuroimaging) have been validated for the diagnosis of anxiety in patients with cognitive impairment.

Treatment. treatment of anxiety disorders ideally requires a combination of psychotherapy and pharmacotherapy, although individual patients may benefit from either one alone, or from a combination of the two. Health care providers will often have to conduct a trial of several different approaches before identifying the optimal treatment strategy. Multiple different therapy modalities are available for the treatment of anxiety, including cognitive-behavioral therapy (effective for all anxiety disorders), exposure therapy (indicated for situational anxiety and specific phobias), and psychodynamic therapy (preferred for patients with milder forms of cognitive impairment).[24] We present a summary of pharmacological agents used for anxiety treatment in **Table 5**.

Apathy

Definition and pathogenesis. Apathy is defined as the absence of interest or initiative to engage with internal and external stimuli. It encompasses behaviors of indifference, unawareness, and lack of concern, emotion, or responsibility. Clinically, apathy has been described predominantly as a motivational impairment and a symptom of various neuropsychiatric illnesses and syndromes such as depression, dementia, and delirium. However, apathy can also occur independently as a syndrome with the above symptoms.[25,26] The limbic pathways connecting the caudate nucleus, internal segment of globus pallidus, and the medial dorsal thalamic nuclei with the prefrontal cortex are most often associated with changes in motivational behaviors. The medial frontal and anterior cingulate circuits are the primary frontal subcortical systems whose dysfunction is relevant to motivational disorders and apathy.[26] Abnormalities in these neural circuits result in dysfunction of dopaminergic, cholinergic, glutamatergic, and monoaminergic transmission–all relevant to the pathogenesis of apathy. Among patients with dementia, apathy severity has been specifically linked to striatal dopamine uptake, whereas lack of initiative has been associated with putamen dopamine transporter uptake.[26–28]

Diagnosis. As for other neuropsychiatric conditions, the diagnosis of apathy can be arrived using a clinical interview, or using validated questionnaires. As part of the diagnostic approach to apathy, it is crucial to determine whether cardinal signs and symptoms (lack of energy, lack of initiative, and amotivation) are present as an isolated syndrome, or in the setting of other disorders (especially depression). Delirium, fatigue, and psychosis can also mimic clinical manifestations of apathy. Health care providers should also elicit a history about medications, with specific emphasis on the use of SSRI (with apathy representing and established side effect). Several self-report and informant questionnaires are available for the diagnosis of apathy, with the most commonly used being the 18-item Apathy Evaluation Scale (AES) and the Starkstein Apathy Scale (SAS).[28,29] There are currently no structured interview tools specifically aimed at diagnosis apathy. At present, no specific biomarkers (serological, in CSF, or neuroimaging) have been validated for the diagnosis of apathy in patients with cognitive impairment.

Treatment. The mainstay of apathy treatment has historically comprised mostly non-pharmacologic approaches, including primarily environmental enrichment and cognitive-behavioral therapy (CBT). Targeted pharmacological treatment options are also available (see **Table 5**), although their use is entirely off-label and lacking in the

Table 5

Pharmacological agents used in treatment of behavioral and neuropsychiatric disorders in patients with cognitive impairment and dementia

Drug Class	Agents	Indications and Treatment Considerations	Dosing Initial	Usual Maximum	Specific Risks	Specific Benefits
Antihistamines	Hydroxyzine	Anxiety (acute treatment) *Avoid in the elderly*	25–50 mg as needed	100 mg as needed	Anticholinergic toxicity Delirium Cognitive slowing	Safer for children, adolescents, and pregnant women.
Antipsychotics	Clozapine	Psychosis, delusions, hallucinations	6.25 mg/day	50 mg/day	Agranulocytosis Potential for extra-pyramidal symptoms	Consider for treatment of Parkinson's disease psychosis
	Olanzapine Risperidone Quetiapine Aripiprazole	Agitation/ Aggression	2.5 mg/day 0.5 mg/day 25 mg/day 2–5 mg/day	10 mg/day 1 mg/day 150 mg/day 15 mg/day	Potential for extra-pyramidal symptoms Increased risk for mortality in dementia patients	
Benzodiazepines	Alprazolam Clonazepam Diazepam Lorazepam	Anxiety (acute treatment) *Short-term use only* *Avoid in the elderly*	0.5–1 mg/day 0.5 mg/day 2–5 mg/day 1–2 mg/day	4–6 mg/day 4 mg/day 40 mg/day 6 mg/day	Falls Cognitive slowing Tolerance Dependence	Fast-acting
Beta-blockers	Propranolol Atenolol	Anxiety Phobias	40–60 mg/day 25 mg/day	160 mg/day 100 mg/day	Symptomatic bradycardia and/ or hypotension	Effective for situational anxiety
Dopamine Receptor Agonists (DRAs)	Rotigotine	Apathy	1–2 mg/day	6 mg/day		Effective in Parkinson's Disease

(continued on next page)

Table 5
(continued)

Drug Class	Agents	Indications and Treatment Considerations	Dosing		Specific Risks	Specific Benefits
			Initial	Usual Maximum		
Cholinesterase Inhibitors	Galantamine Rivastigmine Donepezil	Apathy	8 mg/day 3 mg/day 5 mg/day	16–24 mg/day 12 mg/day 10 mg/day	Cholinergic Toxicity	Effective in Alzheimer's disease
Dopamine Reuptake Inhibitors (DRIs)	Modafinil	Apathy	100 mg/day	200 mg/day	May cause headache	
Dopamine-Noradrenaline Reuptake Inhibitors (DNRIs)	Methylphenidate	Depression Apathy	2.5 mg/day	40 mg/day	Increased risk of cardiovascular disease May cause insomnia	
Monoamine Oxidase Inhibitors (MAOIs)	Phenelzine	Depression Anxiety (social)	15 mg/day	60 mg/day	Dietary restrictions Hyperthermia central nervous system (CNS) depression Withdrawal	
	Rasagiline	Apathy	1 mg/day	1 mg/day		Effective in Parkinson's disease
Mood-stabilizing anticonvulsants	Valproate	Apathy Agitation/ Aggression	250 mg/day	1000 mg/day	Limited evidence for apathy	
NMDA receptor Antagonists	Memantine	Apathy	5 mg/day	20 mg/day		Effective in Alzheimer's disease
Other Anti-anxiety Agents	Buspirone	Anxiety Depression Apathy	15 mg/day	60 mg/day	Slow onset of action	Minimal withdrawal Less sedating

Class	Drug	Indication	Starting dose	Target/max dose	Comments	Considerations
Other Antidepressants	Bupropion	Depression	200 mg/day	450 mg/day	Less sexual side effects than SSRI	Increase in seizure risk at high doses
	Mirtazapine	Depression	15 mg/day	45 mg/day	Weight gain; Somnolence	Concomitant treatment of insomnia
Serotonin Receptor Antagonist and Reuptake Inhibitors (SARIs)	Trazodone	Depression; Anxiety; Apathy; Agitation/Aggression	25 mg/day	300 mg/day	Limited evidence for apathy	Concomitant treatment of insomnia
Serotonin-Norepinephrine Reuptake Inhibitors (SNRIs)	Venlafaxine	Depression (first line); Anxiety; Apathy	37.5 mg/day	225 mg/day	Slow onset of action; Blood pressure elevation; Increased risk of cardiovascular disease	Concomitant treatment of apathy and depression
	Duloxetine		30 mg/day	60 mg/day		
Selective Serotonin Reuptake Inhibitors (SSRIs)	Fluoxetine	Anxiety (first line); Depression (first line)	20 mg/day	60 mg/day	Slow onset of action	Best tolerability profile; May cause/worsen apathy
	Sertraline		50 mg/day	200 mg/day		
	Paroxetine		20 mg/day	50 mg/day		
	Escitalopram		10 mg/day	30 mg/day		
	Citalopram		10 mg/day	40 mg/day		
Tricyclic Antidepressants	Amitriptyline	Anxiety; Depression; Avoid in the elderly	35 mg/day	300 mg/day	Anticholinergic toxicity	Helpful for several other conditions (eg, migraine, neuropathic pain)
	Imipramine		75 mg/day	200 mg/day		
	Nortriptyline		25 mg/day	150 mg/day		

firm-established guiding evidence. Overall, patients and caregivers should be consistently educated about the challenges of apathy treatment, with the absence or partial response being a frequent occurrence.[24,30]

Depression

Definition and pathogenesis. Depression is defined by a combination of feelings of sadness, emptiness, impaired sense of self-worth, and loss of pleasure or interest in daily activities that were previously enjoyable.[31] Depression (with or without concomitant apathy) is the most common neuropsychiatric condition affecting individuals diagnosed with cognitive impairment or dementia (see **Table 1**). The pathogenesis of depression is complex, and only partially understood. Although family, twin, and adoption studies established that depressive disorders are highly heritable, very few genetic risk loci have been identified to date.[32] The monoamine deficiency hypothesis has been at the forefront of depression research; under this framework, impaired mono-aminergic transmission in dopaminergic, serotonergic, and noradrenergic circuits is responsible for the onset and persistence of depressive symptoms.[33] GABAergic and glutamatergic neurotransmitter systems have also been implicated in the pathogenesis of depression.[33] Other evidence, primarily derived from biomarker studies, point to upregulation of CNS inflammatory pathways being associated with depression risk.[34] Finally, degenerative brain structural changes (eg, hippocampal volume loss and microvascular white matter disease) have been linked to depressive symptoms, although the exact mechanism underlying these associations remain poorly understood.[35,36] Additional research has also linked depression risk with personal emotive and psychosocial history, as well as with a variety of environmental exposures.[37] However, the specific relevance of these factors to depression onset and course in patients with cognitive impairment and dementia remains to be elucidated.

Diagnosis. Depression is the most frequent comorbid condition in patients with dementia, posing unique diagnostic challenges.[38] Many of the neurocognitive symptoms associated with depression (impaired attention and executive function, decreased processing speed, reduced capacity for complex tasks) may also be secondary to one or more dementing illnesses. Careful evaluation on the part of providers is therefore required to formulate a correct diagnosis.[9] As for other neuropsychiatric conditions, a variety of questionnaires are available to detect depressive symptoms in clinical practice. The Geriatric Depression Scale (GDS)[39] is one of the most commonly used tools to screen for depression. However, previous studies identified that patients with more severe cognitive impairment may under-report depressive symptoms. Indeed, a mini-mental state examination (MMSE) score below 15 was found to reduce the reliability of the GDS.[40] The Center for Epidemiologic Studies Depression (CESD) scale (in the 10- and 20-item versions) is also frequently used to screen for depression, but may equally underperform in severe dementia cases.[41] As caregivers' input becomes more critical to diagnostic accuracy for patients with severe cognitive impairment, screening tools including informant input, like the Cornell Scale for Depression in Dementia (CSDD),[42] may be preferred. Scores above 12 on the CSDD warrant treatment of depressive symptoms, whereas results between 9 and 12 require close monitoring with a future treatment plan.[43] No specific biomarkers have been validated for the diagnosis of depression in patients with cognitive impairment.

Treatment. Non-pharmacological interventions are usually preferred for the initial treatment of depression in patients with cognitive impairment and dementia. Established evidence indicates that, to be successful, interventions should ideally involve both patients and caregivers.[43] CBT, an evidence-based treatment involving coping skills, relaxation techniques, and stress management training, is best suited for highly motivated patients with milder forms of cognitive impairment.[44] Interpersonal psycho-therapy focuses on individuals' interpersonal stances, role transitions, anguish over losses, and interpersonal skill deficits—and is therefore optimal to address conflicts between patients and caregivers.[44] Problem-solving and supportive therapy focus primarily on identifying stressors and developing solution-based applications to address depressive symptoms. It is particularly helpful to assist those caring for patients with more severe cognitive impairment, especially in terms of executive dysfunction.[44–46] Pharmacological treatment is indicated for refractory depression, or for severe depressive symptoms impacting patients' quality of life and safety. Selective serotonin reuptake inhibitors (SSRIs) are generally preferred as first-line agents, owing to their favorable side effect profile. Treatment should always start at the lowest dose possible and escalated gradually and titrated to clinical symptoms while expecting an 8 to 12 weeks delay in therapeutic response.[47,48] Additional information on pharmacological agents recommended for the treatment of depression in patients with cognitive impairment and dementia is presented in **Table 5**.

Psychosis, Delusions, and Hallucinations

Definition and pathogenesis. Psychosis refers to a group of medical conditions characterized by detachment from reality, resulting in affected individuals displaying culturally abnormal beliefs and behaviors. Delusions and hallucinations are the hallmark symptoms of psychosis, but can also present in isolation as part of primary psychiatric disorder or resulting from CNS injury. Delusions are entrenched dysfunctional beliefs in an alternative reality, that is demonstrably misconstrued and untrue to everyone else in the patient's cultural environment. If prominent mood symptoms, hallucinations, and abnormal motor behaviors are absent the diagnosis of delusional disorder is warranted.[49] Conversely, hallucinations are episodes characterized by perceiving (seeing, hearing, touching, or otherwise feeling) stimuli that are not present to others, typically in the form of either objects or people.[50] Of note, the presence of hallucinations in the absence of altered mental status and other psychosis features (as caused by several recreational drugs) is more appropriately referred to as hallucinosis. Psychosis, delusions, and hallucinations often complicate the course of neurodegenerative disorders and are more prevalent in the later disease stages associated with more severe cognitive impairment. The pathogenesis of delusions is not clearly understood, though dopaminergic projections within fronto-subcortical and frontoparietal networks have been the topic of most investigative studies.[51]

Diagnosis. Identification of delusion and hallucinations is usually based on historical information provided by caregivers, though patients may show symptoms for direct observations as well. The diagnostic approach relies on confirmation of the nature of delusions and hallucinations by a discussion with patients and caregivers, followed by an evaluation of potential confounding factors. In patients with dementia, consistent screening for delirium is critical–given its high prevalence and potential to present with repetitive tangential thought processes (that may be mistaken for delusions) and hallucinations. Quantitative evaluation of the severity of delusional and hallucinatory symptoms is best achieved using informant questionnaires for caregivers, with the NPI being the most widely used instrument.[3]

Treatment. Because of the nature of psychosis symptoms and their higher prevalence among individuals with more severe cognitive impairment, non-pharmacological approaches often are of limited benefit. CBT can be used to address false ideas and beliefs, unreasonable anxiety, and societal and environmental disconnect. Treatment of psychosis usually requires prolonged therapy courses, usually in conjunction with medications and other non-pharmacological interventions. Among these, supportive psychotherapy targeting both patients and caregivers can be critical in helping address dysfunctional beliefs and apprehensions.[52] In terms of pharmacological treatment, antipsychotic agents are considered first-line treatment of the management of psychosis, delusions, and hallucinations. Second-generation antipsychotics are usually selected for use in patients with dementia, owing to their relatively favorable side effect profile.[52] We present detailed information on antipsychotics used to treat psychosis associated with dementia in **Table 5.**

SUMMARY

Diagnosis and treatment of behavioral and neuropsychiatric disorders associated with cognitive impairment and dementia remain a challenging process, with substantial knowledge gaps and limited high-quality evidence. When feasible health care providers should focus on non-pharmacological interventions, involving patients and caregivers and other allied health care professionals (psychologists, therapists, and counselors). Nonetheless, use of pharmacological agents under the supervision of an experienced clinician is warranted in all cases where patients' safety and ability to function are severely compromised.

CLINICS CARE POINTS

- Ensure caregivers receive adequate education in how to properly describe and monitor behavioral and neuropsychiatric symptoms
- Always develop a comprehensive dementia care plan, clearly highlighting for patients and caregivers management goals that are both impactful and achievable
- Ensure patients and caregivers have access to and received education about non-pharmacological interventions to manage behavioral and neuropsychiatric symptoms, from simple everyday strategies to comprehensive approaches including therapeutic counseling and environmental changes
- Medication management of behavioral and neuropsychiatric symptoms requires careful trials and titration of different agents, closely following clinical response as the primary desired outcome

REFERENCES

1. Borsje P, Wetzels RB, Lucassen PL, et al. The course of neuropsychiatric symptoms in community-dwelling patients with dementia: a systematic review. Int Psychogeriatr 2015;27(3):385–405.
2. Fauth EB, Gibbons A. Which behavioral and psychological symptoms of dementia are the most problematic? Variability by prevalence, intensity, distress ratings, and associations with caregiver depressive symptoms. Int J Geriatr Psychiatry 2014;29(3):263–71.
3. Cummings JL, Mega M, Gray K, et al. The Neuropsychiatric Inventory: comprehensive assessment of psychopathology in dementia. Neurology 1994;44(12):2308–14.
4. Inouye SK, Westendorp RG, Saczynski JS. Delirium in elderly people. Lancet 2014;383(9920):911–22.
5. De J, Wand AP. Delirium screening: a systematic review of delirium screening tools in hospitalized patients. Gerontologist 2015;55(6):1079–99.

6. Watt JA, Thompson W, Marple R, et al. Managing neuropsychiatric symptoms in patients with dementia. BMJ 2022;376:e069187.
7. Watt JA, Goodarzi Z, Veroniki AA, et al. Comparative efficacy of interventions for reducing symptoms of depression in people with dementia: systematic review and network meta-analysis. BMJ 2021;372:n532.
8. Watt JA, Goodarzi Z, Veroniki AA, et al. Comparative efficacy of interventions for aggressive and agitated behaviors in dementia: a systematic review and network meta-analysis. Ann Intern Med 2019;171(9):633–42.
9. Press D, Alexander M. Management of neuropsychiatric symptoms of dementia. UpToDate, Waltham, MA Accessed 2014;3(24):20.
10. Dennis M, Shine L, John A, et al. Risk of adverse outcomes for older people with dementia prescribed antipsychotic medication: a population based e-cohort study. Neurol Ther 2017;6(1):57–77.
11. Gill S, Rochon P, Herrmann N, et al. Atypical antipsychotic drugs and risk of ischaemic stroke: population based retrospective cohort study. BMJ 2005;330.
12. Schneider Lon S, Dagerman Karen S. Insel Philip: risk of death with atypical antipsychotic drug treatment for dementia: meta-analysis of randomized placebo-controlled trials. JAMA 2005;294(15):1934–43.
13. Sterke CS, van Beeck EF, van der Velde N, et al. New insights: dose-response relationship between psychotropic drugs and falls: a study in nursing home residents with dementia. J Clin Pharmacol 2012;52(6):947–55.
14. Gerlach LB, Kales HC, Kim HM, et al. Trends in antipsychotic and mood stabilizer prescribing in long-term care in the US: 2011–2014. J the Am Medical Directors Assoc 2020;21(11):1629–35.e8.
15. Vasudev A, Shariff SZ, Liu K, et al. Trends in psychotropic dispensing among older adults with dementia living in long-term care facilities: 2004–2013. Am J Geriatr Psychiatry 2015;23(12):1259–69.
16. Donegan K, Fox N, Black N, et al. Trends in diagnosis and treatment for people with dementia in the UK from 2005 to 2015: a longitudinal retrospective cohort study. Lancet Public Health 2017;2(3):e149–56.
17. Association AP. What are anxiety disorders?. 2021. https://psychiatry.org/patients-families/anxiety-disorders/what-are-anxiety-disorders (Accessed 7 January 2022).
18. Maria Cecilia Freitas-Ferrari JECH, Trzesniak Clarissa, Alaor Santos Filho, et al. Neuroimaging in social anxiety disorder: a systematic review of the literature. Prog Neuro-Psychopharmacology Biol Psychiatry 2010;34(4):565–80.
19. Chand SP, Marwaha R. Anxiety. Treasure Island (FL): StatPearls Publishing; 2022. Available at: https://www.ncbi.nlm.nih.gov/books/NBK470361/.
20. Michelle G, Craske MBS. Anxiety. Lancet 2016;388(10063):3048–59.
21. American Psychiatric Association. Anxiety disorders : DSM-5 selections, xiv. Arlington, VA: American Psychiatric Association Publishing; 2016. p. 114.
22. Cortés N, Andrade V, Maccioni RB. Behavioral and neuropsychiatric disorders in Alzheimer's disease. J Alzheimer's Dis 2018;63(3):899–910.
23. Goodarzi Z, Samii L, Azeem F, et al. Detection of anxiety symptoms in persons with dementia: a systematic review. Alzheimers Dement (Amst) 2019;11:340–7.
24. Orgeta V, Leung P, Del-Pino-Casado R, et al. Psychological treatments for depression and anxiety in dementia and mild cognitive impairment. Cochrane Database Syst Rev 2022;4(4):Cd009125. PubMed PMID: 35466396; PMCID: PMC9035877 not involved in data extraction for this study. AS and MO were principal investigators in one of the included studies, and were not involved in data extraction for this study. There are no other known conflicts of interest.

25. Mann RS. Differential diagnosis and classification of apathy. Am J Psychiatry 1990;147(1):22–30.
26. Chase TN. Apathy in neuropsychiatric disease: diagnosis, pathophysiology, and treatment. Neurotoxicity Res 2011;19(2):266–78.
27. Chong T-J, Husain M. The role of dopamine in the pathophysiology and treatment of apathy. Prog Brain Res 2016;229:389–426.
28. David R, Koulibaly M, Benoit M, et al. Striatal dopamine transporter levels correlate with apathy in neurodegenerative diseases: a SPECT study with partial volume effect correction. Clin Neurol Neurosurg 2008;110(1):19–24.
29. Hum S, Fellows LK, Lourenco C, et al. Are the items of the starkstein apathy scale fit for the purpose of measuring apathy post-stroke? Front Psychol 2021;12. https://doi.org/10.3389/fpsyg.2021.754103.
30. Oba H, Kobayashi R, Kawakatsu S, et al. Non-pharmacological approaches to apathy and depression: a scoping review of mild cognitive impairment and dementia. Front Psychol 2022;13:815913.
31. Wang S, Nussbaum AM, American Psychiatric Association. First edition. DSM-5 pocket guide for elder mental health, ix. Arlington, Virginia: American Psychiatric Association Publishing; 2017. p. 364.
32. Sullivan PF, Neale MC, Kendler KS. Genetic epidemiology of major depression: review and meta-analysis. Am J Psychiatry 2000;157(10):1552–62.
33. Hasler G. Pathophysiology of depression: do we have any solid evidence of interest to clinicians? World Psychiatry 2010;9(3):155.
34. Lotrich FE, El-Gabalawy H, Guenther LC, et al. The role of inflammation in the pathophysiology of depression: different treatments and their effects. J Rheumatol Suppl 2011;88:48–54.
35. Aizenstein HJ, Baskys A, Boldrini M, et al. Vascular depression consensus report - a critical update. BMC Med 2016;14(1):161.
36. Geerlings MI, den Heijer T, Koudstaal PJ, et al. History of depression, depressive symptoms, and medial temporal lobe atrophy and the risk of Alzheimer disease. Neurology 2008;70(15):1258–64.
37. Nemeroff CB. The state of our understanding of the pathophysiology and optimal treatment of depression: glass half full or half empty? Am J Psychiatry 2020; 177(8):671–85.
38. Jones BN, Reifler BV. Depression coexisting with dementia. Evaluation and treatment. Med Clin North Am 1994;78(4):823–40.
39. Pocklington C, Gilbody S, Manea L, et al. The diagnostic accuracy of brief versions of the Geriatric Depression Scale: a systematic review and meta-analysis. Int J Geriatr Psychiatry 2016;31(8):837–57.
40. McGivney SA, Mulvihill M, Taylor B. Validating the GDS depression screen in the nursing home. J the Am Geriatr Soc 1994;42(5):490–2.
41. Logsdon RG, Teri L. Depression in Alzheimer's disease patients: caregivers as surrogate reporters. J Am Geriatr Soc 1995;43(2):150–5.
42. Alexopoulos GS, Abrams RC, Young RC, et al. Cornell scale for depression in dementia. Biol Psychiatry 1988;23(3):271–84.
43. Lyketsos CG, Lee HB. Diagnosis and treatment of depression in Alzheimer's disease. Dement Geriatr Cogn Disord 2004;17(1–2):55–64.
44. Weissman M, Verdeli H. Interpersonal psychotherapy: evaluation, support, triage. Clin Psychol Psychother 2012;19(2):106–12.
45. Espinoza RT, Unützer J, Schmader KE. Diagnosis and management of late-life unipolar depression2. Waltham (MA): UpToDate; 2015. Wolters Kluwer Accessed on August.

46. Areán PA, Raue P, Mackin RS, et al. Problem-solving therapy and supportive therapy in older adults with major depression and executive dysfunction. Am J Psychiatry 2010;167(11):1391–8.

47. Lyketsos CG, DelCampo L, Steinberg M, et al. Treating depression in Alzheimer disease: efficacy and safety of sertraline therapy, and the benefits of depression reduction: the DIADS. Arch Gen Psychiatry 2003;60(7):737–46.

48. Netzel PJ, editor. The physician's guide to depression and bipolar disorders. Mayo Clinic Proceedings. Rochester, MN: Elsevier; 2007.

49. Manschreck T. Delusional disorder. The spectrum of psychotic disorders Neurobiol Etiol Pathogenesis. Cambridge: Cambridge University Press; 2007. p. 116–36.

50. Waters F, Fernyhough C. Hallucinations: a systematic review of points of similarity and difference across diagnostic classes. Schizophr Bull 2017;43(1):32–43.

51. Arciniegas DB. Psychosis. Continuum (Minneapolis, Minn) 2015;21(3 Behavioral Neurology and Neuropsychiatry):715–36.

52. Manschreck TC. Pathogenesis of delusions. Psychiatr Clin North America 1995; 18(2):213–29.

Working Together Globally

Harmonizing Ethno-Regionally Diverse Datasets to Advance the Global Epidemiology of Dementia

Darren M. Lipnicki, PhD[a],*, Ben C.P. Lam, PhD[a],
Louise Mewton, PhD[a], John D. Crawford, PhD[a],
Perminder S. Sachdev, MD, PhD[a,b]

KEYWORDS

- Harmonization • Dementia • Prospective • Retrospective • Integrative data analysis
- Neuropsychological tests • Neuroimaging

KEY POINTS

- Data from multiple sources often represent heterogeneous methodology that includes different assessment instruments and classification criteria.
- Harmonization is the process by which data for similar measures or constructs from different sources are made more comparable.
- Harmonization enables data from multiple sources to be analyzed simultaneously, with techniques such as mega-analysis and individual participant data meta-analyses.
- Statistical harmonization is needed for neuropsychological test data, with methods including standardization, latent variable modeling, and the use of multiple imputation.
- The most popular approach for harmonizing neuroimaging data is ComBaT, with other applications to dementia research including normative modeling and machine learning approaches to statistical harmonization.

INTRODUCTION

Age is the biggest risk factor for cognitive impairment (CI) and dementia, and the global societal and financial burdens these conditions impose are increasing as the world's population ages.[1] Globally, the number of people with dementia is estimated to reach around 150 million by 2050, with the greatest increases expected to occur in developing

[a] Centre for Healthy Brain Ageing, University of New South Wales, Level 1, AGSM (G27), Gate 11, Botany Street, Sydney, New South Wales 2052, Australia; [b] Neuropsychiatric Institute, The Prince of Wales Hospital, Sydney, Australia
* Corresponding author.
E-mail address: d.lipnicki@unsw.edu.au

Clin Geriatr Med 39 (2023) 177–190
https://doi.org/10.1016/j.cger.2022.07.009
0749-0690/23/© 2022 Elsevier Inc. All rights reserved.

regions, including Africa.[1] Research on CI and dementia is lacking in many low and middle-income countries (LMICs).[2] However, the research results from one country or population do not apply to another, with reported differences in the epidemiology of CI and dementia among countries,[3] as well as among different races/ethnicities within countries.[4] Research into how cognitive decline can be slowed and CI and dementia ultimately prevented are thus necessarily a global effort, using large samples with data from different ethno-regions. Resource and coordination limitations mean that data on this scale will typically not come from a single source. Rather, such data must be collated from across multiple unique sources focused on particular countries or regions.

The data needed to understand the epidemiology, cause, and risk and protective factors for CI and dementia comprise a vast array of types, including, but not limited to, demographics, diagnoses, cognitive or neuropsychological test results, medical histories, lifestyle variables such as physical activity, substance use and diet, functional status, neuroimaging, and biomarkers. Each data type can be assessed in many ways, and collaborative efforts that use data from multiple sources are faced with the challenge of making these data comparable, so they can be pooled for analysis or more accurately compared.

In this review, we discuss how data used in dementia and CI research can be made more comparable by harmonization. We cover the benefits and challenges of harmonization, and outline broad retrospective and prospective approaches. We also describe harmonization for particular data types, focusing on neuropsychological test results and neuroimaging, but also including dementia diagnoses, behavioral and psychological symptoms of dementia (BPSD) instruments, and electroencephalography (EEG) measures.

DISCUSSION
What Is Data harmonization? Qualitative and Quantitative Approaches

Harmonization is the process by which data for similar measures or constructs from different sources are made more comparable, or inferentially equivalent.[5] The type of harmonization process needed to achieve comparability depends on the sort of data involved, and may be qualitative or quantitative.

Qualitative approaches lead to data from different sources having a common format, such as the same range of response options or categories, sometimes requiring a transformation process.[6,7] Examples of this approach include the following:

- Choosing an item from each source that best represents the measure or construct of interest, for example, different questions addressing subjective cognitive decline (for a more detailed account, **Box 1**).
- Creating a categorical variable by choosing cut-points for different continuous scales measuring the same construct, for example, classifying the presence of current depression based on a score of 6+ on the Geriatric Depression Scale (GDS) used by one source, and a score of 16+ on the Center for Epidemiologic Studies Depression Scale (CES-D) used by another source (for a more detailed account see Table S11 in Lipnicki and colleagues[8]).
- Collapsing response categories in the data for some sources to make them similar to those for data from another source with fewer response categories, for example, self-rated health scales with different numbers of response categories (**Table 1**).

Quantitative harmonization is needed for more complex data types and often requires statistical processing to bring them to a common format.[9] Statistical

Box 1
Qualitative harmonization of self-experienced decline in cognitive capacity

Subjective cognitive decline (SCD) is self-experienced decline in cognitive ability from a normal level in the absence of objective impairment, and may be the first sign of Alzheimer disease.[64] A recent collaborative research project aimed to estimate the prevalence of SCD in and across international cohort studies of aging.[65] Each study contributing data to the project asked their participants different sets and numbers of questions relevant to determining self-experienced decline in cognitive capacity, requiring the data to be harmonized for more accurate comparison and pooling.

The project used 2 approaches to harmonizing self-experienced decline in cognitive capacity: qualitative and quantitative.

Qualitative: Two authors independently compared all items assessing self-experienced decline in cognitive capacity across the studies, and identified one common item from each that broadly addressed problems or difficulties with memory (see **Table 1**). The original data for these items were transformed to a binary variable indicating the presence or absence of self-experienced decline in cognitive capacity, with any indication of decline in the original responses categorized as "presence."

Study	Item Selected for Qualitative Harmonization	Original Coding
Active Aging	Do you feel you have more problems with your memory than most?	1 = yes, 2 = no
CFAS	Have you ever had any difficulty with your memory? If yes, is that a problem for you?	0 = no, 1 = yes, moderate, 2 = yes, severe
EAS	Compared with 1 year ago, do you have trouble remembering things more often, less often or about the same?	1 = more often, 2 = less often, 3 = about the same
SLASII	Overall, how would you rate your memory or other mental abilities as compared with earlier period of your life (more than 1 year ago)?	1 = much better, 2 = a bit better, 3 = a bit worse, 5 = much worse

Note: Only 4 of the 16 studies included in the project are shown.

harmonization is typically required for data from cognitive or neuropsychological tests, of which there are hundreds that differ on characteristics such as the particular cognitive abilities assessed, and the depth to and mode by which they are assessed.[10] A detailed account of approaches to the statistical harmonization of neuropsychological test scores is given in a later section.

Benefits of Harmonized Data

Harmonization is an often-necessary step before integrative data analysis, in which individual participant level data from multiple sources are analyzed simultaneously. Integrative data analysis techniques such as mega-analysis and individual participant data meta-analyses can overcome some of the limitations associated with single studies or meta-analyses of aggregated study data.[6,9] The benefits of harmonized data thus include the capacity to:

- Pool data from different sources, which increases the sample size and thereby the statistical power:
  - This is particularly important when analyzing rare conditions, characteristics, or outcomes, given the increased absolute numbers of individuals with these (for details, see Hussong and colleagues[6])

Table 1	
Example of self-rated health scale harmonization	
Study	**Coding of Original Response Options to Very Good = 1, Good = 2, Poor = 3**
Bambui	Very Good, Good = 1; Reasonable = 2; Fair = 3
CFAS	Excellent = 1; Good = 2; Fair, Poor = 3
EAS	Excellent, Very Good = 1; Good = 2; Fair, Poor = 3
HK-MAPS	Cumulative Illness Rating Scale sum of various organ system severity ratings: 0,1 = 1; 2–4 = 2; 5–13 = 3
Invece.Ab	Visual analog scale: 0–6 = 1; 7–8 = 2; 9–10 = 1
KLOSCAD	Excellent, Good = 1; Fair = 2; Poor = 3
LEILA75+	Very Good/Excellent = 1; Good = 1; Fair = 2; Poor = 3; Very Poor = 3
MoVIES	Excellent = 1; Good = 2; Fair, Poor = 3
PATH	Excellent, Very Good = 1; Good = 2; Fair, Poor = 3
SALSA	Excellent, Very Good = 1; Good = 2; Fair, Poor = 3
SGS	Very Good = 1; Good = 2; Fair, Poor = 3
SLASI	Excellent, Very Good = 1; Good = 2; Fair, Poor = 3
Sydney MAS	Excellent, Very Good = 1; Good = 2; Fair, Poor = 3

Note. Taken from S9 Table in Lipnicki et al. showing how the original self-reported health data from 13 international cohort studies of aging were harmonized to a 3-category variable representing response options very good, good, and poor.

Adapted from Lipnicki DM, Makkar SR, Crawford JD, et al. Determinants of cognitive performance and decline in 20 diverse ethno-regional groups: A COSMIC collaboration cohort study. PLoS Med. 2019;16(7):e1002853; under CC BY 4.0.

- o Pooling data can similarly increase the number of participants from subgroups that may be typically underrepresented in single studies.[6]
- • Make more accurate comparisons across data sources using measures that are more similar:
  - o This is particularly relevant for investigations of commonalities and differences in factors contributing to CI and dementia across different countries, regions of different economic development, or different races/ethnicities[11] (for examples of relevant research studies, **Box 2**).
- • Conduct validation of results or replication across multiple data sources.[5]

Other benefits associated with harmonization include the opportunity for extended use of existing datasets through collaborative projects where data are shared.[7] Indeed, data sharing has become of increasing importance, with many publishers and funders now encouraging or requiring data sharing, for example, the publishing company Elsevier[12] and the National Institutes of Health, USA.[13]

General Challenges of Data Harmonization

The potential for different data sources to have used considerably different methods to measure the same construct often makes harmonizing data challenging, particularly for cognitive data, given the vast range of tests available.[10] The process can be time consuming and resource intensive,[5] even more so when done on a global scale where translation and cultural differences may need to be considered. It should also be noted that harmonization is often specific to the requirements of a certain research question.[5] Further, transformation of raw data to harmonized data can involve some loss or distortion of information, such as when a variable with 5 response options or

> **Box 2**
> **Using harmonized cognitive impairment and dementia data for international comparisons**
>
> When researching MCI and dementia on a global scale, a great benefit of using harmonized data is the capacity for more accurate comparisons across different ethno-regions.
>
> - *More accurate comparisons of prevalence and incidence of dementia and related conditions.* Although the high variation in reported rates of MCI across different countries is partially explained by differences in location and demographics, there is a significant contribution from differences in definition and methodology.[66] These differences can be reduced by harmonizing cognitive test, functional and subjective cognitive complaint data, and applying a uniform approach to classifying MCI. This approach has yielded much more similar rates of MCI than previously reported.[25] The figure shows the prevalence of MCI previously reported for 7 cohort studies representing 5 different countries alongside more uniform rates produced using harmonized data.[25]
>
>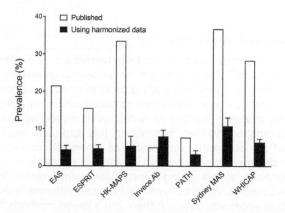
>
> - *Better understanding of risk factors for dementia and related conditions as universal, or as differing between races/ethnicities and regions, including strength of association between risk factors and outcome.* Not only are there ethno-regional differences in the prevalence of risk factors for dementia, such as more diabetes and hypertension in developing countries such as India[2] but analysis of harmonized data on an international scale suggests that the strength of association between particular risk factors and CI and dementia can also differ.[8] A risk factor's prevalence and strength of association with dementia determine the proportion of dementia in a population that can be attributed to the risk factor. This proportion was able to be estimated for various dementia risk factors and more accurately compared across 8 countries where identical 10/66 protocols had been used.[67]

a continuous scale is collapsed to a common format variable with 3 response categories (see **Table 1**).

Retrospective and Prospective Approaches to Data Harmonization

Most of our discussion of harmonization refers to *retrospective data harmonization*, which is applied to preexisting data where constructs or characteristics of interest were obtained or recorded differently by different sources (for an example, see **Box 1**). An alternative approach is *prospective data harmonization*, which is the implementation of uniform protocols across different studies or research centers before data collection occurs, so that data are collected in a harmonized way. Examples of prospective data harmonization on an international scale are the 10/66 dementia research group protocols for addressing dementia epidemiology in Latin America,

China and India,[14] the Harmonized Cognitive Assessment Protocol designed to enhance comparisons across international sister studies of the US Health and Retirement Study,[15] and the Latin America and the Caribbean Consortium on Dementia (LAC-CD), which aims to facilitate comparisons of dementia between countries with harmonized dementia diagnoses.[16] Similarly, prescriptive approaches have been developed for retrospective data harmonization, including a set of guidelines outlining the procedural steps.[5] There have also been attempts to develop systems that facilitate retrospective data harmonization, such as DataSHaPER[17] and the BioSHaRE Project.[18] Full adherence to a harmonized protocol can be compromised by context-dependent requirements, such as the need to replace a cognitive task requiring spelling ability in populations with low rates of literacy.[19] In addition, it has been suggested that the evidence produced by repeated implementation of a protocol across samples may be weaker than evidence from studies using different methodologies.[5]

Harmonizing Neuropsychological Test Data

Neuropsychological test data can be complex to harmonize. There are more than 500 neuropsychological tests[20] and 70 different tests commonly used to assess dementia.[21] A simple method to harmonize such data is to analyze a *common* test or set of tests and treat raw scores as equivalent across sources. In aging research, this has been done for a limited number of widely used measures, such as the Mini-Mental State Examination (MMSE).[22] However, this approach excludes potentially useful studies that do not use the same test(s) as others. Moreover, when evaluating cognition across different ethno-racial populations, it is traditional to base assessments on standardized scores (using appropriate norms) rather than regard raw scores as being equivalent. When different sources use different tests, harmonization requires a statistical approach, of which there are 3 broad methods:[9,23]

- Standardization
- Latent variable modeling
- Use of multiple imputation.

Standardization

Standardized scores can be used to interpret an individual's test performance. Some test manuals present standardized scores (z-scores with a mean of 0 and a standard deviation [SD] of 1) for different demographic groups, defined by sex and ranges of age and/or education. These demographically adjusted standardized scores are the ones most commonly used when neuropsychologists determine diagnoses of mild cognitive impairment (MCI) or dementia. However, when harmonizing test scores across studies from different ethno-racial populations, such manuals are usually not available. In this situation, regression models have been used to produce demographically adjusted standardized scores, using an appropriate normative sample. In community-based longitudinal studies, the baseline sample (excluding those with serious illness or dementia) has been used as the normative sample. Demographically adjusted scores can then be obtained as the standardized residuals in regression models, with demographic variables (usually age, sex, and education) as the independent variables and the raw test scores as the dependent variable. Equations used to obtain these standardized scores at baseline can then be applied to raw scores at later waves to produce scores that are comparable across waves. This method of harmonizing cognitive tests across cohorts has been done previously[24,25] (see **Box 2** for an illustration on harmonizing MCI diagnoses based on standardized cognitive scores).

When research examines the associations of age, sex, and education with cognitive performance, demographically adjusted scores would not serve as the appropriate outcome variables. If analyses are confined to a single study, z-scores with means and SDs calculated using the baseline sample (or other appropriate normative sample) could be used. However, such within-study z-scores would not be comparable across studies owing to their different distribution of demographic characteristics. One solution is to form "demographic category-centered scores" (or C-scores).[9,26] Here, subsamples with the same sex and ranges of age and/or education are selected in each study, and their means and SDs are used to calculate C-scores within each study. For example, subsamples of women aged 70 to 70 years with 8 to 13 years of education were used to harmonize cognitive test scores in 3 Canadian studies.[26] A limitation of this method is the possibility of not obtaining subsamples of sufficient size to reliably estimate the means and SDs required. To overcome this, a modified procedure uses regression models to estimate means and SDs within each study, conditional on common values of the demographics, chosen to be close to the mean or median values across all studies.[27]

Latent variable modeling

Latent variable modeling assumes the existence of latent factors (or constructs) underlying a set of neuropsychological tests or test items (or more generally, observed indicators). Two modeling methods are the use of item response theory (IRT)-based models and linear factor analysis (LFA).

IRT is a framework for understanding the psychometric properties of a test and its items.[28,29] IRT is especially relevant in integrative data analysis[30,31] because it allows the identification of item biases across studies and demographic groupings, referred to as *differential item functioning* (DIF), and it uses tests that are both common and noncommon across studies to estimate the underlying construct (for an illustration of linking see **Box 3**). IRT-based latent variable modeling has been used for harmonizing longitudinal cognitive data.[32] An example of using LFA in structural equation modeling to obtain latent cognitive factors can be found in Salthouse and colleagues.[33]

Box 3
Quantitative harmonization of self-experienced decline in cognitive capacity

The quantitative harmonization approach used both common and unique items to model the latent construct of self-experienced cognitive decline that is equivalent in meaning and metrics across studies.[64] The common item serves as an anchor to link the unique items, for example, item 2 in Study 2 can be linked to item 6 in Study 3 via the common item. The 2-Parameter Logistic IRT model[30,31] was used to evaluate measurement equivalence of the items (item difficulty and item discrimination) across studies, and based on the model, latent scores for each participant were estimated.

	Study			
Items	1	2	3	4
1. Common item (see **Box 1**)				
2. Have you tended to forget things recently?				
3. Difficulty remembering names/things of close people				
4. Difficulty remembering where you kept/put things				
5. More effort to remember things than used to?				
6. In the past year, how often did you have trouble remembering things?				
7. Memory worse than 10 y ago				

Recently, a moderated nonlinear factor analysis model has been developed to handle mixed distributions of observed indicators (eg, binary, ordinal, and continuous).[30] This method has the additional advantages of modeling nonlinear associations between items and the latent factor, and allowing the model parameters to be moderated by categorical (eg, sex, study membership) and continuous (eg, age) covariates simultaneously for testing DIF.

Multiple imputation

Tests or test items that are not assessed in a particular study can be considered as missing by design and handled using statistical models such as multiple imputation. Values for missing items/tests in one study can be imputed using information from items/tests overlapping across studies as well as other related variables in the combined data set but does not require the overlapping items/tests to be in every study. Typically, multiple imputed data sets are generated, and each analyzed separately en route to a pooled estimate. Alternatively, values can be averaged across the imputed data sets to generate a full data set. Burns and colleagues[34] shows how missing MMSE item scores across studies can be imputed and a full data set analyzed.

Harmonizing Neuroimaging Data

MRI data can be valuable for understanding and diagnosing neurodegenerative diseases.[35] The cost and time associated with collecting neuroimaging data mean it is often necessary to combine data collected from multiple sites and across diverse populations and experimental conditions to enhance both statistical power and generalizability of findings. This multisite approach to the collection and analysis of neuroimaging data for dementia research includes the Alzheimer's Disease Neuroimaging Initiative (ADNI),[36] ENIGMA,[37] and CHARGE[38] consortia. A major challenge for pooling multisite neuroimaging is the lack of standardization in both technical aspects (ie, scanner platforms, image acquisition, and processing protocols), as well as differences in sample characteristics (ie, inclusion/exclusion criteria and sample size).[39]

Methods for the prospective harmonization of neuroimaging data in the dementias field have been developed by consortia, multicenter studies and working groups and can include standardization of definitions and frameworks (eg, for imaging of white matter hyperintensities[40]), imaging acquisition protocols (eg, for vascular dementia[41]), and segmentation procedures (eg, for hippocampal volume[42]). Data quality control procedures can also be standardized,[43] whereas containerized software packages can be distributed to ensure consistency in software across sites and time.[44] However, studies have shown that even after careful prospective harmonization, systematic differences in images and sample characteristics across sites may lead to bias in MRI-derived measures.[45] Retrospective data harmonization approaches have therefore been developed that allow the pooling of imaging datasets from heterogeneous sources in an unbiased manner.

One of the most widely used methods for retrospective harmonization of neuroimaging data is the *ComBaT* approach, a technique originally developed to remove batch effects in genomics data.[46] ComBaT was first extended to the harmonization of diffusion tensor imaging data[46] and has recently been applied to the harmonization of structural neuroimaging data in both cross-sectional[39] and longitudinal contexts,[47] as well as functional neuroimaging data.[48] ComBaT corrects for site (or scanner) differences via an empirical Bayes algorithm that estimates and removes location (mean) and scale (variance) differences across sites before downstream analysis. Clinically relevant variations are preserved by defining covariates of interest and incorporating their effect on the variance. ComBaT has been applied to the harmonization of dementia datasets[49] and shown to outperform other site correction techniques.[39]

Other approaches to the harmonization of multisite neuroimaging data include *Neuroharmony*, a supervised machine learning approach that predicts ComBaT correction factors from imaging quality metrics.[50] In a process akin to pediatric growth charts, *normative modeling* uses percentiles to chart the variation of an outcome brain measure normed to the variation of a set of clinically relevant covariates that, in a multisite framework, can include site as a covariate of interest.[51] Recent reviews have identified the potential of this normative approach to address heterogeneity in neuroimaging models of dementia.[52] *Deep learning approaches* have also been developed that are based on generative adversarial networks. These aim to extract a set of imaging features that are maximally informative for an outcome of interest (eg, Alzheimer disease) while also being maximally uninformative about the site or scanner where the data originated.[53] These approaches to the retrospective harmonization of neuroimaging data have their advantages and disadvantages[54] but each has the potential to provide more powerful and generalizable research into neurodegenerative disorders.

Harmonizing Dementia Diagnoses

Autopsy-based diagnoses are the gold standard for dementia and other neurodegenerative diseases. Recent advancements in brain imaging, such as PET scans for amyloid beta and tau, have improved the accuracy of Alzheimer disease diagnoses. However, this is expensive and not always possible for cohort studies of aging, especially in LMICs. Many research studies therefore rely on clinical diagnoses of dementia but there are substantial differences in diagnostic procedures (eg, consensus by an expert panel, assessment tools like the Clinical Dementia Rating scale, the Geriatric Mental State interview) and criteria (eg, DSM-III-R, DSM-IV, ICD-10) across studies.[1,55] These methodological differences can result in varying estimations of dementia rates.[56] Dementia can be diagnosed from assessments of cognitive performance and instrumental functioning, and algorithms derived from these can be a standardized method of dementia classification across studies (see Prince and colleagues[57] for an algorithm developed in the 10/66 project). Recently, an IRT-based model was used to harmonize dementia classifications in 2 cross-sectional studies[58] but its application to a larger number of and more diverse studies has yet to be examined.

Harmonizing Behavioral and Psychological Symptoms of Dementia Instruments

One challenge for the collection and pooling of BPSD data across studies is the large array of available tools that measure the same or similar constructs. In terms of prospective harmonization of BPSD measures, several consensus guidelines have been developed,[59] with many recommending the Neuropsychiatric Inventory for global assessment of BPSD, as well as more specific measures such as the Geriatric Depression Scale and the Dimension Apathy Scale.[59] Many of these recommended tools are available in multiple languages, including those from LMICs.

Quantitative approaches to the retrospective harmonization of BPSD measures also hold great promise for pooling data that have already been collected or when the adoption of consensus guidelines is not appropriate. Harmonization across BPSD measures often necessitates the identification of common items for linking purposes, and this process for BPSD measures has been detailed recently in a reproducible manner.[60] However, when compared with quantitative harmonization of cognitive measures, the application of these approaches to BPSD instruments has been limited.

Quantitative harmonization has been used to develop common metrics, or cross-walks, which link various measures of neuropsychiatric symptoms,[61] although this approach has not yet been initiated in the dementias field.

Harmonizing Electroencephalography Measures

As a low cost and minimally invasive measure of brain connectivity, EEG represents a viable option for measuring dementia biomarkers in LMICs. To encourage multicenter harmonization of EEG data, the Electrophysiology Professional Interest Area and Global Brain Consortium have endorsed recommendations for EEG measures in clinical trials of Alzheimer disease, including for stratification of participants and the monitoring of disease progression.[62] Meanwhile, recent efforts have focused on developing standardized guidelines and best practices for EEG data acquisition, preprocessing, and data analysis that can be applied to multicenter EEG studies of brain connectivity more broadly.[63]

SUMMARY

Dementia research is enhanced by bringing together data from multiple sources. However, methodological heterogeneity means that the data typically need to be retrospectively harmonized, sometimes even when prospective approaches to minimize heterogeneity have been implemented. The particular harmonization methods required depend on the data type, and range from a relatively simple choice of comparable items across sources, to the statistical and technology-driven methods needed to harmonize neuropsychological test scores and neuroimaging data, respectively. Although often a resource intensive process, harmonization can facilitate data pooling and thereby enhance statistical power. Harmonization can also enable more accurate comparisons, such as comparisons of the prevalence and effects of risk factors for dementia across diverse ethno-regional groups.

CLINICS CARE POINTS

- With the increasing digitalization of medical care, data from diverse sources must be harmonized for efficient clinical care and facilitation of clinical research.
- Barriers and facilitators of harmonization should be identified at the national and international levels, so that global clinical research and practice can inform clinical care and prevention of dementia in all jurisdictions.
- Policies and frameworks should be put into place to facilitate harmonization of clinical and research data at both national and international levels.

DISCLOSURE

Dr. Lipnicki received funding from National Institute On Aging of the National Institutes of Health (Award number: RF1AG057531).

REFERENCES

1. GBD 2019 Dementia Forecasting Collaborators. Estimation of the global prevalence of dementia in 2019 and forecasted prevalence in 2050: an analysis for the Global Burden of Disease Study 2019. Lancet Public Health 2022;7(2): e105–25.

2. Ravindranath V, Sundarakumar JS. Changing demography and the challenge of dementia in India. Nat Rev Neurol 2021;17(12):747–58.
3. Prince M, Wimo A, Guerchet M, et al. World Alzheimer report 2015: the global impact of dementia. An analysis of prevalence, incidence, cost and trends. London: 2015.
4. Shiekh SI, Cadogan SL, Lin LY, et al. Ethnic differences in dementia risk: a systematic review and meta-analysis. J Alzheimers Dis 2021;80(1):337–55.
5. Fortier I, Raina P, Van den Heuvel ER, et al. Maelstrom Research guidelines for rigorous retrospective data harmonization. Int J Epidemiol 2017;46(1):103–5.
6. Hussong AM, Curran PJ, Bauer DJ. Integrative data analysis in clinical psychology research. Annu Rev Clin Psychol 2013;9:61–89.
7. Shishegar R, Cox T, Rolls D, et al. Using imputation to provide harmonized longitudinal measures of cognition across AIBL and ADNI. Sci Rep 2021;11(1):23788.
8. Lipnicki DM, Makkar SR, Crawford JD, et al. Determinants of cognitive performance and decline in 20 diverse ethno-regional groups: a COSMIC collaboration cohort study. Plos Med 2019;16(7):e1002853.
9. Griffith L, van den Heuvel E, Fortier I, et al. In: Harmonization of Cognitive Measures in Individual Participant Data and Aggregate Data Meta-Analysis. Rockville (MD): 2013.
10. Briceno EM, Gross AL, Giordani BJ, et al. Pre-statistical Considerations for harmonization of cognitive instruments: harmonization of ARIC, CARDIA, CHS, FHS, MESA, and NOMAS. J Alzheimers Dis 2021;83(4):1803–13.
11. Vonk JMJ, Gross AL, Zammit AR, et al. Cross-national harmonization of cognitive measures across HRS HCAP (USA) and LASI-DAD (India). PLoS One 2022;17(2): e0264166.
12. Elsevier. Available at: https://www.elsevier.com/authors/tools-and-resources/research-data.
13. NIH. Available at: https://sharing.nih.gov/data-management-and-sharing-policy/about-data-management-sharing-policy/data-management-and-sharing-policy-overview#after.
14. Prince M, Ferri CP, Acosta D, et al. The protocols for the 10/66 dementia research group population-based research programme. BMC Public Health 2007;7:165.
15. Langa KM, Ryan LH, McCammon RJ, et al. The health and retirement study harmonized cognitive assessment protocol project: study design and methods. Neuroepidemiology 2020;54(1):64–74.
16. Ibanez A, Parra MA, Butler C, et al. The Caribbean consortium on D. The Latin America and the Caribbean consortium on dementia (LAC-CD): from Networking to research to implementation Science. J Alzheimers Dis 2021;82(s1):S379–94.
17. Fortier I, Burton PR, Robson PJ, et al. Quality, quantity and harmony: the DataSHaPER approach to integrating data across bioclinical studies. Int J Epidemiol 2010;39(5):1383–93.
18. Doiron D, Burton P, Marcon Y, et al. Data harmonization and federated analysis of population-based studies: the BioSHaRE project. Emerg Themes Epidemiol 2013;10(1):12.
19. Torres JM, Glymour MM. Future Directions for the HRS harmonized cognitive assessment protocol. Forum Health Econ Policy; 2022.
20. Lezak MD, Howieson DB, LD W, et al. Neuropsychological assessment. 4th ed. New York: Oxford University Press; 2004.
21. Maruta C, Guerreiro M, de Mendonca A, et al. The use of neuropsychological tests across Europe: the need for a consensus in the use of assessment tools for dementia. Eur J Neurol 2011;18(2):279–85.

22. Gross AL, Sherva R, Mukherjee S, et al. Calibrating longitudinal cognition in Alzheimer's disease across diverse test batteries and datasets. Neuroepidemiology 2014;43(3–4):194–205.
23. Griffith LE, van den Heuvel E, Fortier I, et al. Statistical approaches to harmonize data on cognitive measures in systematic reviews are rarely reported. J Clin Epidemiol 2015;68(2):154–62.
24. Abner EL, Schmitt FA, Nelson PT, et al. The statistical modeling of aging and risk of Transition project: data collection and harmonization across 11 longitudinal cohort studies of aging, cognition, and dementia. Obs Stud 2015;1(2015):56–73.
25. Sachdev PS, Lipnicki DM, Kochan NA, et al. The prevalence of mild cognitive impairment in diverse Geographical and ethnocultural regions: the COSMIC collaboration. PLoS One 2015;10(11):e0142388.
26. Griffith LE, van den Heuvel E, Raina P, et al. Comparison of standardization methods for the harmonization of Phenotype data: an application to cognitive measures. Am J Epidemiol 2016;184(10):770–8.
27. Lipnicki DM, Crawford JD, Dutta R, et al. Age-related cognitive decline and associations with sex, education and apolipoprotein E genotype across ethnocultural groups and geographic regions: a collaborative cohort study. Plos Med 2017; 14(3):e1002261.
28. Bock RD, Gibbons RD. Item response theory. John Wiiley & Sons Inc; 2021.
29. Embretson SE, Reise SP. Item response theory for psychologists. Mahwah (NJ): Erlbaum; 2000.
30. Bauer DJ, Hussong AM. Psychometric approaches for developing commensurate measures across independent studies: traditional and new models. Psychol Methods 2009;14(2):101–25.
31. Curran PJ, Hussong AM, Cai L, et al. Pooling data from multiple longitudinal studies: the role of item response theory in integrative data analysis. Dev Psychol 2008;44(2):365–80.
32. Gross AL, Mungas DM, Crane PK, et al. Effects of education and race on cognitive decline: an integrative study of generalizability versus study-specific results. Psychol Aging 2015;30(4):863–80.
33. Salthouse TA. Localizing age-related individual differences in a hierarchical structure. Intelligence 2004;32(6).
34. Burns RA, Butterworth P, Kiely KM, et al. Multiple imputation was an efficient method for harmonizing the Mini-Mental State Examination with missing item-level data. J Clin Epidemiol 2011;64(7):787–93.
35. Jovicich J, Barkhof F, Babiloni C, et al. Harmonization of neuroimaging biomarkers for neurodegenerative diseases: a survey in the imaging community of perceived barriers and suggested actions. Alzheimers Dement (Amst) 2019;11: 69–73.
36. Alzheimer's disease neuroimaging initiative. 2017. Available at: https://adni.loni.usc.edu/.
37. ENIGMA: Enhancing Neuro imaging Genetics through meta analysis. Available at: https://enigma.ini.usc.edu/.
38. Cohorts for Heart and aging research in genomic epidemiology (CHARGE) consortium. 2022. Available at: https://www.hgsc.bcm.edu/human/charge-consortium.
39. Fortin JP, Cullen N, Sheline YI, et al. Harmonization of cortical thickness measurements across scanners and sites. Neuroimage 2018;167:104–20.
40. Roseborough AD, Saad L, Goodman M, et al. White matter hyperintensities and longitudinal cognitive decline in cognitively normal populations and across

diagnostic categories: a meta-analysis, systematic review, and recommendations for future study harmonization. Alzheimers Dement 2022.

41. HARNESS HARmoNising brain imaging MEthodS for VaScular contributions to neurodegeneration. Available at: https://harness-neuroimaging.org/.

42. Frisoni GB, Jack CR Jr, Bocchetta M, et al. The EADC-ADNI Harmonized Protocol for manual hippocampal segmentation on magnetic resonance: evidence of validity. Alzheimers Dement 2015;11(2):111–25.

43. Samann PG, Iglesias JE, Gutman B, et al. FreeSurfer-based segmentation of hippocampal subfields: a review of methods and applications, with a novel quality control procedure for ENIGMA studies and other collaborative efforts. Hum Brain Mapp 2022;43(1):207–33.

44. Waller L, Erk S, Pozzi E, et al. ENIGMA HALFpipe: Interactive, reproducible, and efficient analysis for resting-state and task-based fMRI data. Hum Brain Mapp 2022;43(9):2727–42.

45. Guo C, Niu K, Luo Y, et al. Intra-scanner and Inter-scanner reproducibility of Automatic white matter hyperintensities Quantification. Front Neurosci 2019;13:679.

46. Fortin JP, Parker D, Tunc B, et al. Harmonization of multi-site diffusion tensor imaging data. Neuroimage 2017;161:149–70.

47. Beer JC, Tustison NJ, Cook PA, et al. Longitudinal ComBat: a method for harmonizing longitudinal multi-scanner imaging data. Neuroimage 2020;220:117129.

48. Yu M, Linn KA, Cook PA, et al. Statistical harmonization corrects site effects in functional connectivity measurements from multi-site fMRI data. Hum Brain Mapp 2018;39(11):4213–27.

49. Eshaghzadeh Torbati M, Minhas DS, Ahmad G, et al. A multi-scanner neuroimaging data harmonization using RAVEL and ComBat. Neuroimage 2021;245:118703.

50. Garcia-Dias R, Scarpazza C, Baecker L, et al. Neuroharmony: a new tool for harmonizing volumetric MRI data from unseen scanners. Neuroimage 2020;220:117127.

51. Marquand AF, Kia SM, Zabihi M, et al. Conceptualizing mental disorders as deviations from normative functioning. Mol Psychiatry 2019;24(10):1415–24.

52. Verdi S, Marquand AF, Schott JM, et al. Beyond the average patient: how neuroimaging models can address heterogeneity in dementia. Brain 2021;144(10):2946–53.

53. Moyer D, Ver Steeg G, Tax CMW, et al. Scanner invariant representations for diffusion MRI harmonization. Magn Reson Med 2020;84(4):2174–89.

54. Bayer JMM, Thompson PM, Ching CRK, et al. Site effects how-to & when: an overview of retrospective techniques to accommodate site effects in multi-site neuroimaging analyses. PsyArXiv Preprints 2022.

55. Prince M, Bryce R, Albanese E, et al. The global prevalence of dementia: a systematic review and metaanalysis. Alzheimers Dement 2013;9(1):63–75 e62.

56. Erkinjuntti T, Ostbye T, Steenhuis R, et al. The effect of different diagnostic criteria on the prevalence of dementia. N Engl J Med 1997;337(23):1667–74.

57. Prince MJ, de Rodriguez JL, Noriega L, et al. The 10/66 Dementia Research Group's fully operationalised DSM-IV dementia computerized diagnostic algorithm, compared with the 10/66 dementia algorithm and a clinician diagnosis: a population validation study. BMC Public Health 2008;8:219.

58. GBD Dementia Collaborators. Use of multidimensional item response theory methods for dementia prevalence prediction: an example using the Health and Retirement Survey and the Aging, Demographics, and Memory Study. BMC Med Inform Decis Mak 2021;21(1):241.

59. Costa A, Bak T, Caffarra P, et al. The need for harmonisation and innovation of neuropsychological assessment in neurodegenerative dementias in Europe: consensus document of the Joint Program for Neurodegenerative Diseases Working Group. Alzheimers Res Ther 2017;9(1):27.

60. Chen D, Jutkowitz E, Iosepovici SL, et al. Pre-statistical harmonization of behavioral instruments across eight surveys and trials. BMC Med Res Methodol 2021; 21(1):227.

61. Batterham PJ, Sunderland M, Slade T, et al. Assessing distress in the community: psychometric properties and crosswalk comparison of eight measures of psychological distress. Psychol Med 2018;48(8):1316–24.

62. Babiloni C, Arakaki X, Azami H, et al. Measures of resting state EEG rhythms for clinical trials in Alzheimer's disease: recommendations of an expert panel. Alzheimers Dement 2021;17(9):1528–53.

63. Prado P, Birba A, Cruzat J, et al. Dementia ConnEEGtome: towards multicentric harmonization of EEG connectivity in neurodegeneration. Int J Psychophysiol 2022;172:24–38.

64. Jessen F, Amariglio RE, van Boxtel M, et al. A conceptual framework for research on subjective cognitive decline in preclinical Alzheimer's disease. Alzheimers Dement 2014;10(6):844–52.

65. Rohr S, Pabst A, Riedel-Heller SG, et al. Estimating prevalence of subjective cognitive decline in and across international cohort studies of aging: a COSMIC study. Alzheimers Res Ther 2020;12(1):167.

66. Ward A, Arrighi HM, Michels S, et al. Mild cognitive impairment: disparity of incidence and prevalence estimates. Alzheimers Dement 2012;8(1):14–21.

67. Mukadam N, Sommerlad A, Huntley J, et al. Population attributable fractions for risk factors for dementia in low-income and middle-income countries: an analysis using cross-sectional survey data. Lancet Glob Health 2019;7(5):e596–603.

Moving?

Make sure your subscription moves with you!

To notify us of your new address, find your **Clinics Account Number** (located on your mailing label above your name), and contact customer service at:

Email: journalscustomerservice-usa@elsevier.com

800-654-2452 (subscribers in the U.S. & Canada)
314-447-8871 (subscribers outside of the U.S. & Canada)

Fax number: 314-447-8029

Elsevier Health Sciences Division
Subscription Customer Service
3251 Riverport Lane
Maryland Heights, MO 63043

ELSEVIER

Printed and bound by CPI Group (UK) Ltd, Croydon, CR0 4YY

03/10/2024

01040471-0001